# Swindon College

## GNVQ Advanced Options

## Human Physiology and Health
## in the Caring Context

GNVQ Advanced Options

# Human Physiology and Health in the Caring Context

Sue Ford • Ann Richards
Eileen Asiedu-Addo • Anna Maidwell

*Redwood College of Health Studies,*
*South Bank University, London*

STANLEY
THORNES

© Sue Ford (Chapters 5 and 6), Ann Richards (Chapters 1, 3 and 7), Eileen Asiedu-Add (Chapters 2 and 7) and Anna Maidwell (Chapters 4 and 7) 1995

Published in 1995 by
Stanley Thornes Publishers Ltd
Ellenborough House
Wellington Street
Cheltenham
GL50 1YW
UK

97 98 99 00 01 / 10 9 8 7 6 5 4 3

A catalogue record for this book is available from The British Library.

ISBN 0 7487 1770 6

Typeset by Stanley Thornes (Publishers) Ltd
Printed and bound in Great Britain

# Contents

# Introduction

This book has been compiled to support students studying for the Advanced GNVQ in Health and Social Care. The chapters have been compiled to reflect the content of the optional units covering human physiology and health offered by BTEC, City and Guilds and RSA.

The content is broadly based upon the elements, performance criteria and range statements of each unit. Each chapter includes Activities designed to capture the interest of the student, promote the use of a problem-solving approach and present opportunities for the development of evidence for inclusion in the student's portfolio. Care points, to emphasise the application of the theoretical perspectives to practice, are also scattered throughout the text.

In addition, self-assessment sections called Twenty Questions at the end of each chapter enable the student to test their knowledge and understanding. Chapters are concluded by a section of Quick Concepts which review key terms and issues discussed in the preceding pages (key terms are in bold type the first time they occur).

Although the book has been written for the GNVQ student, it is also intended to be of general value to anyone working in the care sector. The authors hope that all readers, whether studying predominantly theoretical perspectives or gaining practical workplace experience will find illumination and inspiration and a fuller understanding of the rewarding fields of health and social care.

Sue Ford
Ann Richards
Eileen Asiedu-Addo
Anna Maidwell

Redwood College of Health Studies
South Bank University, London, 1995

# Acknowledgements

The authors and publishers would like to thank the following people and organisations for permission to reproduce photographs and other material:

George Montgomery/Photofusion (page 90); Rob Scott/Photofusion (page 96); Vania Coimbra/Photofusion (page 97); John Libbey & Company Ltd for the chart on page 63; Pictor International Ltd for the cover photograph.

Every effort has been made to contact copyright holders and we apologise if any have been overlooked.

# 1 Control mechanisms in the human body

## What is covered in this chapter

- The construction of living things
- Body cells and their structure
- The genetic code
- Homeostasis
- Communication and control systems
- Hormonal control of body function
- The nervous system
- Two neurological diseases

## Introduction

Life began in the sea with tiny, one-celled creatures whose internal body composition closely resembled the water that they lived in. There was no problem maintaining a constant internal environment because it closely matched the external environment. All their nutrients, oxygen and body fluids were obtained by the simple process of **diffusion** into their one cell. Diffusion is the passage of molecules from an area of high concentration to one of lower concentration. A one-celled creature that lives today is an amoeba, a tiny animal that lives in fresh water. If there is more oxygen in the water than in an amoeba, diffusion of oxygen will occur from the water into the cell. Waste products, such as carbon dioxide, will pass, by diffusion, out of the cell where there is a high concentration.

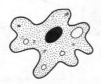

*A simple one-celled organism: the amoeba*

As animals with many cells developed there had to be specialised **tissues** for obtaining and transporting oxygen and nutrients around the body and eliminating waste. Simple diffusion is too slow a process to operate over distances larger than one or two cells.

## Activity 1.1

Try to think of the systems that have developed to obtain and transport oxygen and nutrients around the body.

Examples of some systems that have evolved are:
- the respiratory system to obtain oxygen
- the digestive system to obtain nutrients
- the circulatory system to transport the oxygen and nutrients to all cells.

The development of all these different systems means that the human body is composed of trillions of cells with thousands of chemical processes occurring each second.

## The construction of living things

A living thing capable of a separate existence is called an **organism.** In a simple one-celled creature there is only one cell to do everything. As creatures developed with more cells it became necessary for different cells to adopt different functions. As the body became larger, some sort of transport system was necessary to ensure that nutrients and oxygen reached all areas. This transport system is the blood, and the cells in the blood have become very specialised, some to transport oxygen – the red cells – and others to help combat infection – the white cells.

The process by which cells become specialised is called **differentiation** and it is vital to the functioning of the human body.

### Examples of differentiated cells

| Type of cell | Function |
| --- | --- |
| A nerve cell | Conduction of impulses |
| A red blood cell | Transport of oxygen |
| An egg cell | Reproduction |
| A muscle cell | Contraction |
| A gland cell | Secretion |

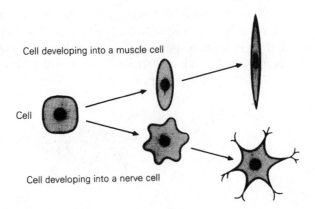

*Cell differentiation*

Groups of cells of the same type make up the different tissues of the body; for example, muscle tissue is made up of muscle cells, all packed closely together. Several types of tissue together form an **organ**; for example, the stomach is an organ made up of muscle tissue, epithelial tissue and connective tissue. An organ has a specific job to do. The liver is the busiest organ in the body and has over 500 functions. A number of organs together form a system; for example, the digestive system is made up of the gut, the pancreas, the liver and the gall bladder. These organs all work together to digest and absorb the food eaten.

# Body cells and their structure

Although cells are highly differentiated, all animal cells have certain common features:

- They are surrounded by a membrane, which allows certain substances such as water and nutrients to pass into the cells but is not freely permeable to all substances.
- They have a control centre called the **nucleus**: it is inside the nucleus that the genetic material is kept. This holds the pattern for the manufacture of all the different types of **protein** in the cell and acts as a blueprint for the replication of the cell. The genetic material is held in a highly specialised substance called **DNA** (Deoxyribonucleic acid).
- The cell is filled with **cytoplasm**: this is a jelly like substance in which the chemical reactions of the cell can take place.
- Inside the cell are **organelles**: these are tiny bodies in cytoplasm. There are several types of organelle, each with its own function, for example ribosomes are organelles that manufacture protein; **mitochondria** are the 'powerhouses' of the cell and extract energy from glucose.

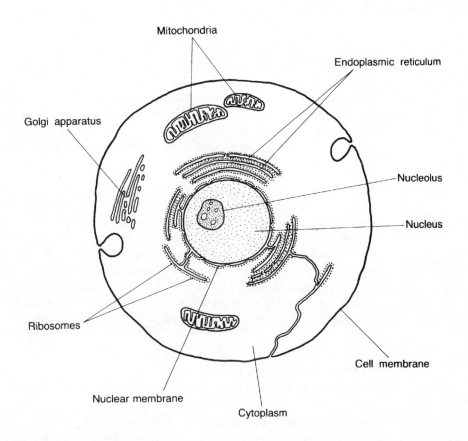

*A typical animal cell*

## Cell division

Cell division is the splitting up of one cell (the parent cell) into two cells (daughter cells). The two daughter cells are identical to the parent cell. This type of cell division is called **mitosis**. Cell division is necessary to replace worn out body cells, but it is also needed for growth to occur. Growth is an increase in size that occurs as an organism develops.

Human life starts off as a single cell: the fertilised egg. This single cell divides into two cells, then four, then sixteen and so on. The illustration below shows what happens when a cell divides. The daughter cells are smaller at first, but soon increase to the size of the parent cell.

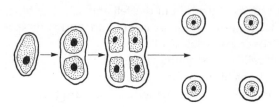

*Cell division*

## Growth and differentiation

When the embryo has reached the size of about 20 cells, cells begin to change shape and differentiation starts to occur. The type of cell they turn into depends on their position in the organism; for example, if a cell is in the head, it may become a brain cell.

In a growing child cell division is occurring all over the body and the child increases in size. Not all parts of the body grow at the same rate, however; the head grows quickly at first then slows down, whereas the limbs grow slowly at first and speed up later. Growth stops when no more cells are added to the body. In humans this occurs at about the age of 18.

**Care point**

A growing child needs a balanced diet, to provide the ingredients necessary for the manufacture of new cells. New tissue is mostly made up of protein which is therefore an essential constituent of the diet. However, many of the processes involved in cell division and growth also require small amounts of vitamins. One example is folic acid, one of the vitamin B group. This vitamin is essential for cell division to occur correctly. Although a balanced diet is needed at all ages, it is very important that the growing child has all the nutrients it needs. As we get older we do not need to replace as many body cells and can survive if necessary on a diet of poorer quality.

### The importance of protein

- Proteins form much of the structural component of the body, for example the muscles.
- Any tissue that is specialised is made up of protein.
- Many important secretions are made of proteins. This includes the **hormones** which are chemical messengers and are discussed in more detail later. Secretions

also include **enzymes** which are biological **catalysts** and are essential for the chemical reactions that are constantly occurring in the body.

The body manufactures protein from amino acids which it obtains from the breakdown of protein in the diet.

# The genetic code

The nucleus of the cell contains the DNA (see above, page 3). DNA contains the genetic code, or blueprint for the manufacture of every protein in the body. If anything goes wrong with the DNA the wrong proteins will be made. This is the cause of many genetic disorders. One example is sickle cell anaemia where one wrong amino acid is put into the haemoglobin of the red cell, which alters the shape of the red cell; because of this the cells are broken down too quickly, making the person anaemic. Anaemia is present when there is insufficient haemoglobin in the blood.

## Chromosomes

The DNA in the nucleus is contained in the genes. The genes are the units of heredity and are carried on the **chromosomes.**

A person has 23 pairs of chromosomes in each cell nucleus. One of each pair has come from their mother and one from the father. A picture of the 23 pairs of chromosomes is called a karyotype and is shown below.

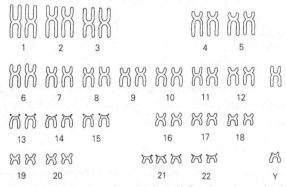

The chromosome pattern of a male infant with Down's syndrome, showing the extra number 21 chromosome, Trisomy 21

*The human karyotype consisting of 23 pairs of chromosomes*

In certain genetic disorders there may be an extra chromosome. One example here is trisomy 21 or Down's syndrome. Instead of having two number 21 chromosomes, the baby has three.

It is the extra genetic material on this chromosome that causes the typical features of Down's syndrome: slanting eyes, rounded face, a flat nasal bridge and short stature.

## Activity 1.2

A chromosomal disorder such as Down's syndrome will have many effects on the child, both physical and psychological, as well as far reaching effects on the family as a whole. Identify the physical effects on a baby of trisomy 21 by referring to a genetics textbook. Now think about the influence of these on the child as they grow up and also on the family. Look at psychological and social effects as well as physical. (You can obtain extra information to help you with this task from the Down's Syndrome Association, 12 Clapham Common Southside, London SW14 7AA.)

# Homeostasis

The essential chemical processes in the body cells are controlled by enzymes which are biological catalysts made of protein. Enzymes can only operate within narrow temperature and acidity ranges. This means that the internal environment of the cell must be kept relatively constant to maintain normal body function. Maintaining a stable internal body temperature of about 37 $^0$C when the outside environment is continuously changing, is **homeostasis.**

To maintain this stability of environment in each cell, there has to be a good system of communication throughout the body. If a child is hungry, it will ask for food. This is communication. Similarly, if cells do not have enough glucose for energy they have to ask for more. (In this example, the extra glucose may come from the liver, an organ which can release glucose from its energy stores). This communication in the body involves the nervous system (page 15) and the hormones (see page 9).

## Maintaining homeostasis

The balancing process required to maintain homeostasis involves three functional parts:
• receptors
• a control centre
• a responding organ.

Receptors monitor the internal environment. They pass their information to the control centre which initiates the correct response by sending out nervous or hormonal messages to the responding organ.

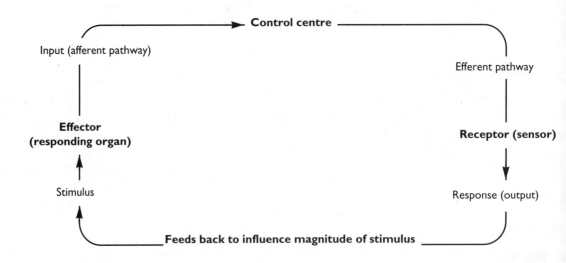

*An example of homeostatic feedback*

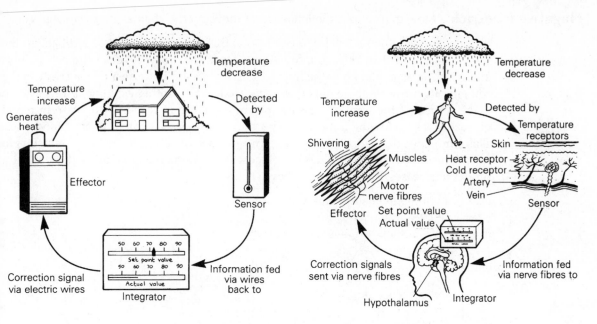

*A heating system as an example of negative feedback*     *The feedback control of temperature in the body*

This regulation can be compared to the central heating system in a house (above left). Most chemical processes in the body are controlled by this process of negative **feedback**. The nerve endings in the skin are the receptors that monitor temperature. If the temperature rises they send a nervous impulse to the brain, the control centre. The brain then sends a message to the sweat glands and stimulates them to function. Evaporation of the sweat causes cooling and homeostasis is restored (above right).

## Feedback mechanisms in the human body

When the body is in homeostasis the needs of its cells are being met and all is functioning smoothly. If homeostasis is disturbed this results in an imbalance which may have serious consequences for the cells. Every body system has some part to play in the maintenance of internal constancy.

# Communication and control systems in the human body

The nervous system is the body's main communication network and is a system of control as well as communication. It works closely with the endocrine system which produces chemical messengers called hormones. These systems regulate the body's responses to the internal and external environment. The messages relayed by the nervous system are very fast, whereas those sent via the chemical messengers take longer to produce change in the body.

## Activity 1.3

Make a list of the body systems you know and write down the part they play in maintaining homeostasis.

## Negative feedback

If, for example, glucose level in a cell is low, this information will be fed back to the liver which will then release more sugar. Once the sugar level in the cell is high enough a message will go to the liver to stop its release. Because a rise in sugar in the cell inhibits further release, this is *negative* feedback. Another example of this system is the release of the hormone insulin by the pancreas in response to a rise in blood glucose levels following a meal. After a meal the glucose content of the blood rises. This stimulates the pancreas to release and produce insulin, the action of which is to reduce the blood glucose. When the glucose level in the blood is lowered the insulin production ceases. This process is shown below.

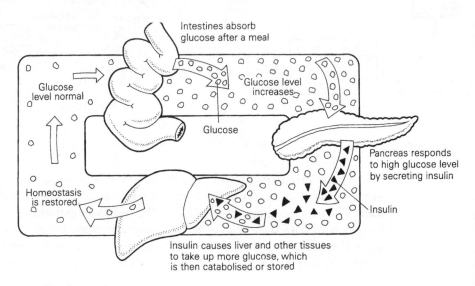

*The control of insulin secretion*

<table>
<tr><td>**Care point**</td><td>In clients with diabetes mellitus there is insufficient insulin production and this means that the glucose in their blood is at too high a level. Some of this glucose spills over into the urine and we can see if someone is diabetic by testing their urine. This is a simple test and may be done in hospital or in the community. A person with diabetes mellitus is taught to test their own urine.</td></tr>
</table>

## Positive feedback

Positive feedback is much rarer in the human body; it occurs when the response to a hormone causes more release of the same hormone. This results in a cascade effect. One example is the stretching of the uterus in labour which stimulates production of oxytocin by the pituitary gland. The oxytocin causes more contraction of the uterus and stretching so that even more oxytocin is produced. This continues until the baby is born.

**Activity 1.4**

The heating system in your house is controlled by negative feedback. Can you think what would happen if it were a positive feedback system instead?

Positive feedback systems are much more likely to go out of control and so are only rarely used in the body, where stability of internal environment is all important. If your central heating was a positive feedback system, when the thermostat was switched on more heat would be produced; this would stimulate the boiler to produce even more heat and the room would get hotter and hotter. There would not be a steady temperature.

Maintenance of a constant internal environment is vital to the health of the body. Some doctors think of the disease process as a change in homeostasis. As ageing occurs, the body becomes less efficient and control of the internal environment becomes more difficult. This means that elderly people are more susceptible to disease processes.

One example is hypothermia, a body temperature below 35 $^0$C. If a young person is in a cold environment their body will produce more heat and their temperature will stay at about 37 $^0$C. The body of an elderly person may not detect the fall in temperature outside and may not respond to increase its temperature. The body temperature may fall to a dangerously low level.

It is very important that the elderly are kept warm and that their houses or other accommodation are not allowed too severe a drop in temperature in the winter. This is an important point in the community where the older person may be trying to economise on heating bills.

# Hormonal control of body function

The endocrine system is a system of ductless glands whose secretions are called hormones. Hormones are released directly into the bloodstream from the **endocrine gland** and have their effect on distant target sites. (This is different from the other type of gland in the body which is called exocrine and does have a duct. A salivary gland is an exocrine gland; it releases its secretion which travels to the mouth via a duct. The saliva then has an effect in the mouth itself. It lubricates the food and starts the digestion of starches. )

The secretion of an endocrine gland does not act near the gland itself but travels in the bloodstream to its target cells. For example, the adrenal gland, which releases adrenaline, is situated on top of the kidney, but the adrenaline works on distant sites such as the heart and the lungs.

## The endocrine glands

There are six main endocrine glands in the body:
- the pituitary gland
- the thyroid gland
- the parathyroid glands
- the adrenal glands
- the pancreas
- the gonads, i.e. ovaries or testes.

Secretions of these glands are controlled mainly by negative feedback. Certain diseases are caused by under- or over-secretion; some of these are mentioned below.

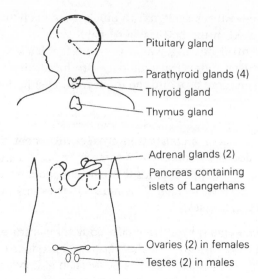

*The endocrine glands*

The endocrine system and the nervous system are not entirely separate entities; there is a small area of the brain called the hypothalamus that helps to maintain homeostasis and provides the link between the nervous system and the endocrine system. The hypothalamus exerts control over the master gland of the body: the pituitary gland.

## The pituitary gland

The pituitary is a small gland the size of a pea. It is situated at the base of the brain and is attached to the hypothalamus by a short stalk. It is often called 'the leader of the orchestra' because it exerts control over many of the other endocrine glands. (Disease of the pituitary gland affects other endocrine glands because they need its stimulating factors.) The pituitary produces more hormones than any other endocrine gland and is divided into two lobes, the anterior lobe and the posterior lobe.

### The anterior lobe

Three hormones are produced by this part of the pituitary:

- growth hormone, produced mainly in childhood. Excess of this hormone leads to gigantism; a deficiency leads to dwarfism. (If a child is deficient in growth hormone this can now be made using genetic engineering and given by injection)
- melanocyte-stimulating hormone, which affects the melanocytes; these produce melanin, a pigment that colours the skin
- prolactin, which is produced after the birth of a baby and stimulates milk production.

These hormones are called stimulating hormones as they stimulate other glands – the adrenals, the thyroid and the gonads – to produce their own secretion.

### The posterior lobe

This part of the pituitary produces only two hormones:

- antidiuretic hormone, which concentrates the urine. More is produced when the body needs to conserve water, for example on a very hot day if sufficient fluids are not taken in. Alcohol prevents the release of this hormone. This means that after an alcoholic drink we produce more urine than normal. If quite a lot of alcohol is consumed this could lead to slight dehydration which is partly responsible for the headache that is part of a hangover next day! This piece of knowledge should give you a clue how to prevent the headache occurring!

- oxytocin causes contraction of the uterus in labour. Oxytocin release was the example given on page 8 to illustrate a positive feedback system. It also controls the release of milk during suckling.

### The thyroid gland

This gland is situated in the neck, spanning the trachea. The hormone it produces is called thyroxin and controls the body's metabolic rate. Metabolic rate is the rate that the body releases energy and this controls the body's level of activity. Some people have higher metabolic rates than others and they tend to be more active, use up more energy and stay slimmer. To produce thyroxin the thyroid needs an adequate supply of iodine in the diet.

   If the thyroid is overactive the symptoms include:

- loss of weight
- increased appetite
- always feeling hot even in cool weather
- fast pulse – even while sleeping.
- hyperactivity – the person finds relaxing difficult
- an alert mind
- insomnia
- tremor.

If the gland is under-active, the reverse of the above symptoms will occur. Under-activity of the gland is sometimes called myxoedema and is more common in the elderly, especially women. It may often be that an elderly client with hypothermia has an under-active thyroid gland. If this is the case, treatment in the form of thyroxin tablets taken daily can return the metabolic rate to normal levels.

---

**Case study**

Mrs Jones, aged 83, complained of feeling cold even in the summer. She said her memory seemed to be getting worse and friends noticed her mind was less agile. She put on quite a lot of weight but insisted she was eating less than she used to. Relatives said she had become rather sluggish and her level of activity had fallen. One morning, after a very cold night in winter, Mrs Jones was found by her daughter sitting in a chair, staring into space and feeling very cold. The ambulance was called and on arrival at hospital Mrs Jones' temperature was 33.5 $^0$C.

This case is typical of many that occur in a cold winter. Elderly clients are admitted to hospital with hypothermia. Great care has to be taken to raise the temperature slowly. On investigation, the thyroid is often found to be under-active and the client is treated with thyroxin tablets.

---

**Care point**

Hypothermia brings extra complications to the elderly. Circulation will be sluggish and this means the client is at more risk of developing pressure sores. Care workers must ensure that if the patient is in bed they are turned from side to side every two hours to prevent pressure sores.

### The parathyroid glands

There are four of these small glands embedded in the four poles of the thyroid gland. They produce parathormone, which maintains the blood calcium at the correct level.

If too much parathormone is produced, calcium is taken from the bones to increase the blood levels beyond normal. The excess calcium in the blood is then excreted by the kidneys and may become deposited in them as stones. These are called renal calculi and are very painful. If too little parathormone is produced, a condition known as tetany results and the muscles go into spasm.

## The adrenal glands

There are two of these glands, one on top of each kidney, rather like a small cap. They are divided into an outer part called the cortex, and an inner part called the medulla, both of which produce their own hormones.

### The adrenal cortex

The adrenal cortex produces:

- steroid hormones, the most important of which is cortisol, which is essential to life. It is important in helping the body to cope with the everyday stresses of life, although scientists still do not understand exactly how it works. Cortisol has anti-inflammatory properties and suppresses the immune system. This has led to its use as a medication in disease where inflammation causes the symptoms, for example asthma. It is also used when we wish to suppress the immune response, as in auto-immune diseases (see page 49) such as rheumatoid arthritis.
- aldosterone is also produced by the adrenal cortex and helps to regulate the sodium and potassium balance of the body. This is more fully described in Chapter 3 when the kidneys are discussed.

### The adrenal medulla

Adrenaline is produced by the adrenal medulla to prepare the body for activity. It is important in the fight, fright and flight response. In other words it prepares the body for any of those three solutions to an emergency and because of this is released at times of acute fear or anger.

## Activity 1.5

Think of a time when you were either very nervous, had a sudden fright or shock or were very angry. The response of your body to these different situations would be similar. Write down the physical effects of the situation on your body. (One example could be the effect on your heart rate.) You should have quite a long list. When you have checked your list against the one given below, think of the reasons behind each effect. Consult a textbook of physiology if necessary.

Adrenaline prepares the body for activity and all its effects on us are towards this end. The effects of adrenaline on the body are to increase the following:

- the speed and force of the heartbeat
- the rate and depth of respiration
- the amount of glucose in the blood
- perspiration.

Adrenaline will cause the following to dilate:

- the bronchioles, allowing more air entry to the lungs
- the blood vessels to skeletal muscle
- the blood vessels to the heart and lungs
- the blood vessels to the brain
- the pupil of the eye.

The following may be constricted:
- the blood vessels to the skin – making the skin feel cold
- the blood vessels to the gut – this may even cause nausea.

### The pancreas

The pancreas is situated in the abdomen and is an exocrine as well as endocrine gland. Its exocrine secretions are **enzymes** released into the duodenum that help to digest our food. In this section we are concerned only with its endocrine function. The pancreas produces two hormones: insulin, which lowers the blood glucose levels and glucagon, which has the opposite effect and raises them.

### Lack of insulin: diabetes mellitus

The release of insulin from the pancreas is dependent on the levels of glucose in the blood. After a meal these will be raised and insulin is released. The insulin enables the glucose in the blood to pass into the body cells and be used for energy. If there is too much glucose, insulin allows the body to store the excess as fat. Without insulin the body cannot utilise glucose which accumulates unused in the blood. As the glucose level gets higher, some of it is excreted by the kidneys in the urine. This is the condition of diabetes mellitus. It is treatable by the administration of insulin by injection throughout life.

Whatever client group you care for, you will always meet some clients with diabetes mellitus. If a person becomes diabetic when they are young it is very likely that they will need to have insulin therapy. Some people who develop diabetes later in life do produce some insulin and can control the diabetes by changing their diet or by taking tablets which stimulate insulin production by the pancreas.

### Glucagon

Glucagon is the other hormone released by the pancreas. It is released when the blood glucose levels are low; for example, if you do not eat any breakfast in the morning, your body still needs glucose for energy. Glucagon will be released and will raise glucose levels by taking sugars from storage.

---

**Case study**

Mrs Thomas, 76, is rather overweight. Over the last few months she has noticed that she is passing more urine and drinking rather more fluids. She is also complaining of itching around the vulva. When her urine is tested glucose is present. (The itching around the vulva is called pruritis and is a common feature of diabetes in the elderly.) The doctor seeing Mrs Thomas will order a blood glucose test which will show an abnormally high level if diabetes is present.

Some general practitioners run their own diabetic clinics and treat their patients either alone or in partnership with the diabetic consultant at the hospital.

---

**Activity 1.6**

Using your knowledge of nutrition and referring to a nursing text if necessary, outline the changes in diet you think would be needed for a client with diabetes. Return to this activity after you have read Chapter 4, *Food, Diet and Nutrition* and revise your plan.

---

### Complications of diabetes

The extra glucose in a person with diabetes can lead to certain complications which mostly affect the blood vessels in different parts of the body. These complications include:

- higher risk of heart disease
- higher risk of stroke
- poor circulation to the legs and feet
- loss of sensation especially in the feet
- kidney damage
- damage to the retina of the eye.

These complications are likely to occur whether the diabetes is insulin-dependent or less severe. They do not start to occur until about fifteen years after the person has become diabetic. It is believed that the better controlled the diabetes, the less likely the complications. Diabetes is well controlled when the blood glucose level is kept as near normal as possible.

**Care point**

One of the most important aspects of long-term care of the person with diabetes is care of the feet. There may be poor circulation and lack of sensation, and if the diabetic damages their foot, even by careless cutting of toe nails, gangrene may develop, which has been known to result in amputation of the foot. This illustrates the importance of health education in diabetes and the need for the elderly diabetic to be visited by the chiropodist to have their nails cut professionally.

### Gonads

Gonads are the ovaries in the female and the testes in the male. They produce sex hormones necessary for the normal development of the body at puberty.

### Female hormones

The main female hormones are called oestrogens, but the ovaries also produce progesterone:

- oestrogens give a woman a different bodily shape from a man and are responsible for breast development at puberty. Scientists also believe they are partly responsible for the reduced risk of coronary artery disease in women. Oestrogen is also needed for the absorption of calcium by the body. After the menopause women's bones may become too brittle due to lack of calcium. This is called osteoporosis and is responsible for the much higher percentage of elderly women than men who break their hips. Hormone replacement therapy in the form of oestrogen and a little progesterone is now taken by many women when they reach the menopause. This should cause a decline in osteoporosis in this group.
- progesterone is especially important in pregnancy.

Oestrogen and progesterone are secreted in different amounts during the menstrual cycle, which they regulate. The secretion of oestrogen falls at the menopause.

### Male hormones

The male hormones are called androgens and include testosterone. Androgens are responsible for the muscular development of a young man as well as the body hair distribution and the deepening of his voice. Male hormones are also needed for the production of sperm.

# Control of endocrine secretion

The secretions of some of the endocrine organs are regulated directly by feedback mechanisms; for example insulin is secreted in response to a high blood glucose. Others, such as cortisol, are regulated by the pituitary, which is in turn influenced by the hypothalamus.

### The hypothalamus

The hypothalamus is part of the brain and is the link between the endocrine system and the nervous system.

- It is only small but is vitally important in the control of homeostasis.
- It controls the output of some hormones.
- It is the centre for control of body temperature.
- It regulates eating behaviour according to levels of nutrients and hormones.
- It regulates thirst, and if body fluids are too concentrated the person will feel thirsty.

*Care point* ▶ The hypothalamus is one of the last areas of the brain to mature. This explains why premature babies are not able to maintain their body temperature without artificial support.

# The nervous system

Consider the following situations:

- you are driving along your normal route home when a dog runs across the road in front of you – you swerve and break to avoid it
- you are busy studying with the radio on for background. You are not listening to it until suddenly one of your old favourites is sung – you immediately hear the song and start to listen
- you are sitting doing the crossword and puzzle hard and long over an evasive clue until you suddenly have the answer.

What do all these actions have in common? They are all examples of how your nervous system deals with everyday life. It is constantly buzzing with activity, and even when you are asleep it will be alert to unusual activity or noise.

The nervous system is the major controlling and communication system of the body. Although it works alongside the endocrine system in the maintenance of homeostasis, it is far more sensitive, fast acting and complex. There are three main functions of nervous tissue:

- the sensory nerves monitor changes in the environment; these changes are called stimuli
- these changes are interpreted and decisions made as to what action needs to be taken; this is called integration
- a response occurs – the contraction of muscles or the stimulation of glands. This is a motor response.

# The central nervous system

The brain and spinal cord make up the **central nervous system** and are the control centres of the body. The brain has been compared to a telephone exchange with messages

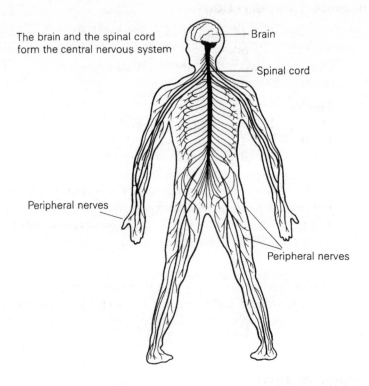

The brain and the spinal cord
form the central nervous system

Brain

Spinal cord

Peripheral nerves

Peripheral nerves

*The central nervous system*

from all over the body being transported to it and relayed from it. It has also been compared to a computer: when the messages arrive the brain interprets them and decides on what action to take.

## The peripheral nervous system

### Sensory nerves

Sensory nerve fibres travel to the brain bringing information from all over the body. Some fibres are sensitive to temperature, some are sensitive to touch, others are sensitive to pain. The sensory fibres in the eye are sensitive to light and those in the ear respond to vibrations.

### Motor nerves

Travelling away from the brain to our muscles are motor fibres. These carry messages away from the brain to the muscles and control body movement. This control is conscious, that is we are aware of what we are doing.

### The autonomic nervous system

Another part of our peripheral nervous system is automatic and based on reflex action. We are not usually conscious of its effects and have very little, if any, control over it. This is called the **autonomic nervous system**. Nerve fibres of the autonomic system go to and from the gut and control its movement. They control the rate of secretion of many glands as well as the acid secretion in the stomach. They also regulate our heart rate and control our blood pressure.

The autonomic nervous system is very important in the maintenance of homeostasis. It keeps our internal environment constant while our external environment is always changing.

The autonomic nervous system has two opposing parts: the sympathetic and the parasympathetic nervous system. Normally there is a balance between the two systems. In an emergency, or when the body is preparing for action, the sympathetic nervous system takes over.

### The sympathetic nervous system
The effects of the sympathetic nervous system are:
- increased heart rate and force
- increased breathing rate and depth
- dilated bronchioles in the lungs
- increased sweating
- dry mouth.

Even without any more effects listed you will probably realise where you have seen these effects before: they are those given by the hormone adrenaline.

The sympathetic nervous system works in much the same way as adrenaline. Its action is more immediate, however, and does not last as long. The sympathetic nervous system stimulates the adrenal glands to produce adrenaline which then prolongs the above actions. This may happen in an emergency such as an accident, when a person is very frightened or in a lot of pain. If blood has been lost, the action of the sympathetic nervous system raises the blood pressure and helps to combat shock. You may have noticed that if someone is in a state of shock or in a lot of pain they feel cold and clammy – a sure sign that the sympathetic nervous system is dominant. Their pulse rate will be increased and their breathing faster than normal.

### The parasympathetic nervous system
This part of the autonomic nervous system is in control when the body is relaxing – perhaps after dinner, sitting in an armchair. The effects of the parasympathetic nervous system are:
- to slow down the heart rate
- to steady the breathing
- to increase peristalsis and secretion of enzymes in the gastro-intestinal tract
- to increase secretion of acid by the stomach
- to allow the body to get on with its everyday activities, such as digesting the food just eaten.

The autonomic nervous system works with the endocrine system to maintain our internal environment in a steady state. It does this without us being aware of all the changes it is constantly making. We may only become aware of its action when we are anxious, for example, and feel our heart thumping away in our chest.

*Care point*

In old age the autonomic nervous system becomes less efficient. Constipation is more common, due to lack of peristalsis in the gastrointestinal tract. The eyes may become dry as less blinking may lead to more frequent eye infections.

## Reflex action

- A **reflex** is a rapid automatic response to a stimulus.
- It does not have to be learned, is not premeditated and is involuntary.
- The same stimulus always causes the same motor response.
- Reflexes are usually protective.

An example of a reflex is that if you touch a hot iron you will withdraw your fingers rapidly and without thinking about it; you will blink if an object approaches your eye. These reflexes are triggered by the spinal cord without any help from the brain, so we do not have to think about them. Some reflexes can be overriden: if you picked up a hot object you would normally let it go, but if the hot object was a very expensive plate then you might well hold on to it!

Doctors test some reflexes to see if the nervous system is functioning adequately. An example is the 'knee jerk' where a tendon hammer is used to tap the area just below the knee and the lower half of the leg is automatically raised upwards.

**Care point**

> Reflexes slow down slightly in old age. An elderly person's response is slower in certain situations. This could affect driving ability, for instance, where we are relying on learned reflex actions the whole time and have to respond rapidly to our environment.

## Nerve cells

Nerve cells are called neurones and are very specialised for the transmission of electrical messages. They use up a lot of energy and need a constant supply of oxygen and glucose from the blood. They cannot survive for more than a few minutes without oxygen. This fact has an implication for carers: if, in a resuscitation attempt, the circulation is not re-established within three minutes, neurones will die and permanent brain damage will result.

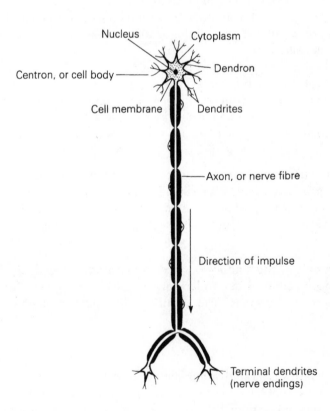

*A nerve cell or neurone*

**Care point**

In difficult childbirth a temporary lack of oxygen to the brain may lead to cerebral palsy, a condition displaying poorly controlled or paralysed muscles. In addition, about half the victims have seizures and half have learning difficulties. Cerebral palsy, which affects six out of every 1000 births, does not deteriorate with time but its effects are permanent. Those working with disabled children will be very familiar with its effects as it is the commonest cause of severe disability in children.

Neurones are not replaceable if destroyed, but with good nutrition can live and function well for at least a hundred years. However, the brain reaches its maximum weight in the young adult and for the rest of our lives neurones are damaged and die and the brain weight decreases. Fortunately the lost neurones are only a very small percentage of the total and there should be very little change in thinking powers in the healthy until the age of 70 or well beyond.

**Care point**

When caring for the elderly it must be understood that there may be some deterioration in short-term memory, but that many other powers function well. The elderly have a wealth of past experience which can still be used, and verbal fluency does not usually decline with age. Fewer than 5 per cent of those over the age of 65 exhibit true senility (loss of intellectual faculties). Carers should beware of making the frequent mistake of forgetting that most elderly people are rational intelligent adults.

## The cerebral hemispheres

The part of the brain that is responsible for our conscious thought is called the cerebrum. It is divided into two halves: the cerebral hemispheres. Each half has several lobes all with their own functions. This part of the brain is awesome in its complexity and staggering in its flexibility of thought. Some functions of the cerebrum are:
- maintaining consciousness
- integration of information
- memory and learning
- speech
- language processing
- personality
- perception, that is interpretation of vision, hearing and situations
- movement
- interpretation of feelings
- control of emotions.

# Two neurological disorders

## The physiological basis of nervous disorders

We have seen how complex the nervous system is. There are very many diseases that may affect it. The older we are, the less able the body is to maintain homeostasis under pressure and the more likely we are to succumb to system breakdown. The symptoms of disease will depend on which part of this complex system is affected.

Two common neurological disorders are briefly described below: Parkinson's disease and Alzheimer's disease.

## Parkinson's disease

Parkinson's disease is a very common disorder in the elderly and care workers in a residential home for the elderly will be bound to meet those with this disease. There is a gradual deterioration of brain cells that produce the chemical dopamine. This chemical has a major effect on movement and Parkinson's disease has two main symptoms: tremor and rigidity. More detailed symptoms are given in the following case study.

---

**Case study**

Mr Grange is 74 years old. Five years ago he noticed a tremor in his right hand. This was very embarrassing for him and he kept his hand in his pocket as much as possible to hide it. The tremor gradually became worse and started to extend to his other arm and hand. Mr Grange went to see his doctor who diagnosed Parkinson's disease. As time progressed Mr Grange also noticed that he was having difficulty with fine movements such as fastening buttons, and that he was becoming more rigid in his walking style.

Although the tablets the doctor gave him seemed to help a little, the symptoms increased in intensity and relatives noticed that Mr Grange's speech was changing and his voice was losing expression. They also noticed that the tremor had spread to his face and could be seen sometimes as a twitch. However, at this time he could carry on with his life and was quite independent.

With the passage of time Mr Grange's walk became more of a shuffle. He had a stooped appearance and a tendency to fall over easily. The stiffness of his muscles began to affect his face, which appeared expressionless. He found talking difficult and could not be easily understood. At mealtimes he was embarrassed because he found chewing difficult and was drooling a lot. As his mobility decreased and he became more frustrated, his wife could no longer manage at home and Mr Grange is now in an elderly persons' home.

---

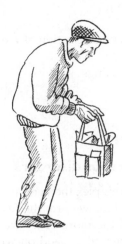

*Stooping posture and shuffling gait are two of the physical signs of Parkinson's disease.*

> **Care point**
>
> Mr Grange in the case study may appear not to communicate, but this is not because he does not wish to. His thinking ability is very likely to be completely unaffected by the disease; Mr Grange has an active mind which is trapped inside an uncooperative body. When caring for people with Parkinson's disease we must always remember this. It can be very difficult to listen to their very slow speech and great patience is needed.

## Alzheimer's disease

Alzheimer's disease is a degenerative condition which is progressive. There is an atrophy (shrinking) of the brain where plaques become deposited in the cerebral cortex. There is loss of memory and behaviour may change. Judgement, intellect and emotional stability are also usually affected. Alzheimer's is the commonest cause of dementia (loss of cognitive function) in this country and the cause is still not known. It is a very tragic disorder, especially for the family of those affected, for they have to watch a loved one's behaviour changing out of all recognition.

## Twenty questions

1   What is differentiation; why did it become necessary when multicellular creatures evolved?

2   Draw an animal cell and label the parts.

3   Why is protein so important in the body?

4   How many chromosomes are there in human cells?

5   What are the two main communication systems of the body?

6   Draw a simple diagram to show any negative feedback system in the body.

7   What is a positive feedback system? Give one example in the body.

8   Name four hormones produced by the anterior pituitary gland.

9   What does the thyroid gland control?

10   What is the name of the disorder when the pancreas is unable to produce enough insulin?

11   Why is hypothermia more of a problem for elderly than younger people?

12   Where are the female hormones oestrogen and progesterone produced?

13   What is the hypothalamus?

14   What are the three main functions of nervous tissue?

15   What two organs make up the central nervous system?

16   Describe the autonomic nervous system.

17   Name six effects that the parasympathetic nervous system has on the body.

18   What is a reflex action?

19   What is Alzheimer's disease?

20   Describe the symptoms of Parkinson's disease.

# Quick concepts

| | |
|---|---|
| **Autonomic nervous system** | Part of the nervous system responsible for the control of bodily functions that are not consciously directed |
| **Catalyst** | A substance that speeds up a chemical reaction while remaining unchanged itself |
| **Central nervous system** | The brain and spinal cord |
| **Chromosome** | A threadlike structure in the cell nucleus that carries genetic information in the form of genes |
| **Cytoplasm** | Jelly like substance that fills the cell |
| **Differentiation** | The process during which cells become specialised to perform a certain function |
| **Diffusion** | The passage of molecules from an area of high to lower concentration |
| **DNA (Deoxyribonucleic acid)** | Genetic material which controls the synthesis of proteins in the body and controls heredity |
| **Endocrine gland** | A ductless gland that releases hormones directly into the blood stream |
| **Enzyme** | A biological catalyst that speeds up the rate of chemical reaction inside the cell |
| **Feedback system** | A system where input is fed to a control centre which then regulates the output. The output is then fed back to the control centre |
| **Homeostasis** | The maintenance of the internal environment of the body in a steady state, even when the external environment is changing |
| **Hormone** | Chemical messenger released by an endocrine gland |
| **Hypothalamus** | A small area of the brain that has many regulatory functions and helps to maintain homeostasis |
| **Mitochondria** | Small organelles (qv) inside the cell that extract energy from nutrients |
| **Mitosis** | Cell division in which a parent cell divides to form two identical daughter cells |
| **Nucleus** | Part of the cell that contains the genetic material |
| **Organ** | Part of the body composed of more than one tissue but functioning as a whole |
| **Organelle** | A small structure found inside the cell, e.g. mitochondria; literally means 'little organ' |
| **Organism** | Any living thing; some are unicellular and consist of only one cell; others are multicellular and may consist of many, many cells |
| **Protein** | Essential constituent of the body, necessary for growth and repair of tissues and regulation of function |
| **Reflex** | An automatic or involuntary activity |
| **Tissue** | A collection of cells specialised to perform a certain function |

# 2   Equilibria systems

## What is covered in this chapter

- Fluid in the body
- The role of the kidneys in maintaining fluid balance
- Temperature regulation
- Control of acidity

## Introduction

The knowledge and application of anatomy and physiology helps the individual to develop an understanding of how the human body works and the changes that may occur as a result of disease or of normal response to the external environment. The body is made up of cells which together form tissues. These tissues are made of essential substances required to maintain their structure and function. Water is one of these substances.

## Fluid in the body

### Proportions

The amount of water as a percentage of the total body weight varies with age and the amount of fat tissue. The more fat present in the individual, the lower the water content. In infants under two years, water makes up 75 per cent of the total body weight; the proportion decreases to about 60 per cent in the adult, and less in an elderly person. It is important for care workers to be aware of these variations and to monitor fluid loss in children and older people and prevent serious complications.

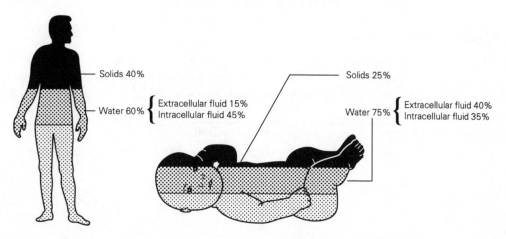

Solids 40%

Water 60% { Extracellular fluid 15%
Intracellular fluid 45%

Solids 25%

Water 75% { Extracellular fluid 40%
Intracellular fluid 35%

## Activity 2.1

Make a list of conditions in a) children and b) older people where fluid may be lost more rapidly than normal.

## Fluid compartments in the body

Fluid is found inside the cells (**intracellular fluid**) and also surrounding them (**extracellular fluid**). Water in intracellular fluid enables chemical reactions to take place within the cells so that health is maintained. All tissues and body fluids contain water. Body fluids outside the cells are divided into tissue fluid, **lymph** and blood. Extracellular fluid provides a constant environment for the cells and a means of transport to and from them.

There is water in secretions of the **gastrointestinal tract,** secretions which enable the breakdown of food into substances that can be used by the body and also in secretions of the joints that facilitate their movement.

In a healthy person there is a constant balance in the amount of water in these fluid compartments. Some people need to have accurate recordings of fluid that enters and leaves the body.

**Care point**

A person who complains of painful joints may have a sample of fluid requested for examination. This investigation may be useful in the diagnosis of inflammatory conditions such as rheumatoid arthritis. Blood present in the fluid may suggest injury to the joint or the condition of haemophilia.

## Sources of water

The body obtains its water supply through fluid and food we ingest, and through **metabolism**, the process by which food is made suitable for the body to use. The rate of metabolism is influenced by age, as is the rate at which water is produced via this method. The metabolic rate is higher in children as their energy demands are greater than those of adults. The metabolic rate in the older person is lower as energy demands decline with age. This is an important consideration when advice about diet is included in any health promotion activities.

## Routes of water loss

Excess water together with end products of metabolism leave the body through sweat, breathing, urine and faeces. The average fluid lost from the different routes of the body of a healthy adult amounts to approximately 2400 ml daily, as shown in the table below.

| Organ | Fluid loss (ml) |
| --- | --- |
| Lungs | 350 |
| Skin | 450 |
| Faeces | 200 |
| Kidneys | 1400 |
| | 2400 |

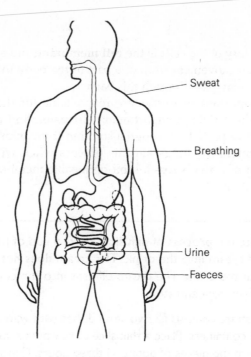

*Routes of water loss*

A balance between the intake and output of water in the body is controlled by certain mechanisms to preserve a constancy in fluid volume. For example, if we drink less water than the body requires, the thirst centre in the brain responds to the low water volume and we experience a sensation of thirst. This will also happen if excess fluid is lost in **diarrhoea** or vomiting. At the same time the kidneys excrete less urine in an attempt to conserve fluid in the body. If this situation persists, water is extracted from the cells and **dehydration** develops.

If we drink more water than the body requires, the excess is largely excreted by the kidneys in the urine and we observe an increase in the volume of urine passed. If fluid accumulates in the tissues, this leads to **oedema**.

## Uses of water

Water acts as a method of transport for some substances in the body. Water, salts and waste products pass backwards and forwards between the blood, tissue fluids and cells. Some of these substances separate or dissociate in water and are called **electrolytes**. Examples of electrolytes are sodium, calcium and potassium.

The concentration of these electrolytes plays a part in the transfer of water between fluid compartments and the cells. Each fluid compartment contains different electrolytes which must remain in their correct solutions if the body is to maintain a constant internal environment (**homeostasis** – see Chapter 1).

*Care point* ▶ A patient may be prescribed drugs to remove excess fluid from the body. These drugs are called diuretics and may be used in heart conditions to encourage the kidney to excrete more fluids.
Electrolytes dissolved in the body fluid may also be lost and can be replaced at the same time intravenously (inserting a hollow tube, a *cannula*, into a vein).

## Water transport

The boundary of the cells is the **cell membrane** and acts as a barrier to certain solutes so that their movement from one part of the body to another is restricted. Water and some salts may pass through this barrier.

Two important processes are responsible for the transfer of water and solutes between the cellular compartments: **diffusion** and **osmosis**. Diffusion involves the movement of particles through a solution from an area of high to low concentration. Oxygen enters the lungs via this process when we breathe in air. Osmosis is the movement of water across a semi-permeable membrane to an area of highly concentrated solution.

### Activity 2.2

To illustrate the process of diffusion, make a cup of black coffee and pour a small amount of cream into the drink. The cream does not stay in one place, but spreads throughout the drink. The cream diffuses into the coffee. It is passing from an area of high to lower concentration.

To demonstrate osmosis fill two small dishes with water. Add two tablespoons of salt to one of the containers. Place a thin slice of raw potato into each container and observe the change in the pieces of potato in three hours. Can you explain this change?

You could do the same experiment using a wilted lettuce leaf instead of a potato – again, explain your results.

## The role of the kidneys in maintaining fluid balance

The kidneys play a major role in the amount of water, electrolytes and waste products lost from the body in the urine.

The kidneys are two bean-shaped organs which lie one either side of the spinal cord. In an adult they measure 10–12 cm (4–5 in) long, 5–7.5 cm (2–3 in) wide and 2.5 cm (1 in) thick. They are enclosed in a capsule and surrounded by a mass of fatty tissue – the adipose capsule which protects them from injury and helps to secure them in place. The kidneys play a major role in the amount of water and waste products lost from the body in the urine.

How does a kidney carry out this function? The kidneys are made up of very small tubules called **nephrons**. Nephrons are divided into a cup-like structure (the Bowman's capsule) and renal tubules. The Bowman's capsule contains a network of capillaries which is branched from the renal artery. These capillaries form what is called the glomerulus. The renal tubules are divided into the proximal tubule, the Loop of Henle, the distal tubule and the straight collecting tubule.

These tubules filter the blood which passes through them so that the amount of substances in the blood are controlled. (The rate of filtration reaches the maximum capacity when a child is between one and two years of age.)

Essential substances are reabsorbed into the blood and waste products remain in the urine. The kidneys remove waste products such as **urea** which is made from protein breakdown. Urea is poisonous and if it was allowed to accumulate in the blood would eventually lead to death.

The filtering of the blood mainly depends on the glomerular blood hydrostatic pressure – the blood pressure in the glomerulus, which averages about 60 mmHg.

The hydrostatic pressure is the force that a fluid under pressure exerts against the walls of its container.

Reabsorption of sodium, potassium and almost all amino acids takes place in the proximal tubule. Regulation of sodium and potassium in response to the body's needs takes place in the Loop of Henle and calcium and magnesium are absorbed in the distal tubule. The remaining fluid passes down the ureters to the bladder to be excreted as urine. Certain factors outside the kidneys influence them in the amount of fluid they reabsorb or eliminate in the urine to preserve constancy in the internal environment of the body. Reabsorption of water by the kidneys is controlled by a hormone secreted by the pituitary gland. It is called **antidiuretic hormone**. This hormone is produced when the body needs to conserve water. It causes less urine, which is more concentrated, to be passed.

Water lost by the kidneys is also affected by the amount of waste product to be lost. There is always a certain amount of metabolic waste to be excreted, although the amount produced depends partly on dietary habits.

If there is an increased amount of waste products to be excreted, the kidneys may require more water to eliminate them. For example, if we eat large portions of chocolate or sugar-containing foods, so that the level of blood sugar vastly exceeds the normal amount, a greater volume of water will be excreted in order to eliminate the sugar. This accounts for the increased urinary output and excessive thirst characteristic of **diabetes mellitus** (see Chapter 1).

The amount of sugar and salt lost from the body is balanced by another hormone produced by the adrenal glands. This is **aldosterone**, and retains the level of sodium in the body at the expense of potassium loss.

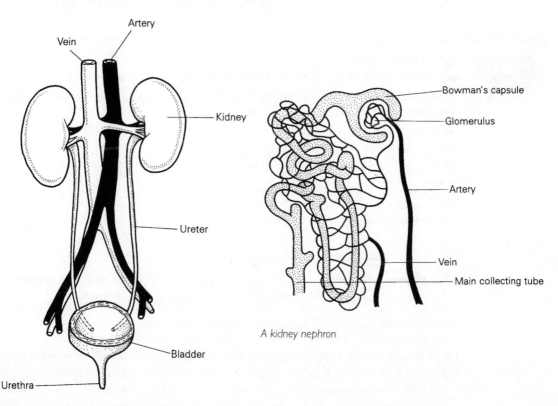

*A kidney nephron*

*The urinary tract*

## Regulation of the internal environment

Some substances are too large to pass through the kidney tubules and therefore remain in the blood. Plasma proteins and blood cells come into this category.

The whole blood volume passes through the kidneys so that waste products are continually being removed. This helps to regulate the body's internal environment so that it remains in constant balance.

## Fluid loss in the urine

About 1.5 litres of urine is passed in 24 hours. However, this volume may vary depending on how much fluid is lost from the body in other ways. Children lose fluids more rapidly than adults as their kidneys do not conserve water as readily. This is an important consideration when children develop conditions that lead to an increase in their body temperature which in turn results in excess fluid being lost via the skin.

The minimum volume of urine needed to excrete waste products is 500–600 ml daily. This amount must be passed even if the body is dehydrated, or the toxic waste would build up in the blood. Normal urine is composed of 96 per cent water and 4 per cent solutes such as urea.

## Kidney disease

If the kidneys are damaged, the substances that are too large normally to pass through their tubules may be able to do so and will then appear in the urine. In the condition acute **glomerular nephritis** the urine may contain protein. The presence of protein in the urine can be checked by testing a urine sample with special reagents.

**Activity 2.3** ───────────────────────────────────────────────

### Daily fluid intake

As shown in the table on page 24, 2400 ml of fluid is lost daily from the different routes in the body. We need to maintain a balance in fluid volume and take in a sufficient amount to replace the lost fluid.

To demonstrate an average fluid intake for yourself, make a list of all the drinks you have in 24 hours. Your intake may follow the pattern shown below, but these volumes may vary from day to day as appetite and exercise levels fluctuate.

| Drinks | 1500 ml |
|---|---|
| Water in food | 700 ml |
| Water from metabolism | 200 ml |
| | 2400 ml |

(The fluid requirements of children are based on their body weight. A new-born infant would require 60–100 ml per kg of body weight in 24 hours.)

---

**Case study**

The following case history will enable you to discuss the problems that a client may have with fluid balance and how you might deal with these problems.

Howard Sinclair, aged 81, is a resident in an old people's home. He suffered a mild stroke six weeks ago, which has left him with weakness down the left side of his body and generally unable to carry out independent self-care activities. He is experiencing particular difficulties with dressing and feeding himself and is anxious to restore a normal or as near normal lifestyle.

Discuss the problems Mr Sinclair will have in maintaining his fluid levels and suggest ways in which these problems can be minimised.

# Temperature regulation

Changes in the weather obviously affect the environment in which we live. If we are to survive these environmental temperature changes, the body has to be able to control its temperature range within the limits that maintain the health of its tissues. A cold-blooded animal such as a tortoise, for example, hibernates in winter because its body temperature adopts the temperature of the external environment.

# Temperature control

Body temperature needs to be controlled because some activities of the body cells are regulated by protein compounds sensitive to temperature. These protein compounds are **enzymes** and they function within a narrow temperature range. The ideal temperature for these enzymes to work is between 36.6–37 $^0$C (98.4–98.6 $^0$F), the normal body temperature.

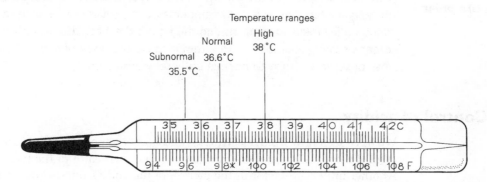

*A clinical thermometer showing subnormal, normal and high temperature*

There may be variations in temperature taken in the morning and the evening. This variation depends on a balance between how much heat the body produces and how much is lost.

# Production of heat in the body

Heat is produced in the body through different activities necessary for the maintenance of life. Two of these activities are the breakdown of food and the movement of muscles.

### Breakdown of food

During the breakdown of food, heat and energy are produced by the organs that take part in these processes. A large amount of heat is produced by the **liver** which is responsible for many metabolic processes.

### Exercise

Contraction of muscle that allows us to move around our environment also produces heat. Heat is continuously being produced and needs to be removed from the body to maintain a constant temperature range for the cells to survive.

The body gets rid of excess heat via the skin using four methods:

- **radiation**
- **conduction**
- **convection**
- **evaporation.**

### Heat loss after exercise

Muscular activity produces heat which needs to reach the surface of the body to be lost via the skin. The blood vessels dilate (widen) to increase the flow of blood which carries excess heat to the skin surface. Heat radiates from the skin to the surrounding air, which has a cooler temperature.

If we sit on a chair the heat from the surface of the body comes into contact with it. Heat is then lost by direct contact. This is conduction. When warm air next to the skin rises and is replaced by cooler air, this is convection.

**Care point**

When someone has a high temperature, a fan may be used to encourage heat loss from the body by convection.

The sweat glands also increase their production to encourage heat loss. In this case heat is lost from the skin as sweat evaporates and cools the body.

In certain infections, the body temperature increases in response to the activity of the invading micro-organisms and the body's defence. You may observe the ill client sweating profusely in an attempt to rid the body of excess heat; then you may observe a return to normal body temperature.

# Control of acidity

We have seen how fluid, electrolytes and body temperature contribute to the constancy of the body's internal environment so that the health of the tissues is maintained. Another important factor in the control of the body's internal environment is the **pH** (acidity/alkalinity) of the body fluids.

## Sources of acids and bases

The food we eat consists mainly of carbohydrates, proteins and fats. These foods have to be broken down into smaller compounds so that they can be used by the body.

Some foods contain **bases** or alkalis and others contain **acids**. Acids come mainly from the production of hydrogen ions in the breakdown of food. If these acids were allowed to accumulate in the food, they would change the environment of the cells and affect chemical activities in the cells or the cell boundaries or membranes. Enzymes (proteins that control chemical reactions of the cells) are sensitive to the amount of acid present and would work less effectively in an acidic environment.

The body has therefore to regulate the concentration of hydrogen ions. It does this with three mechanisms, involving the lungs, the kidneys and the ability of some substances dissolved in the body fluids to restrict or **buffer** other substances so that the pH does not vary widely.

To understand buffering, consider what happens to a mop after you have mopped up water with it. The mop soaks up the water which can be squeezed out and disposed of at a convenient time. A buffer is a substance that soaks up excess acid or base but does not actually dispose of it. The acid or base can be eliminated at a convenient time.

The term pH measures the concentration of hydrogen ions in solution and indicates the degree of acidity or alkalinity of the solution. It is indicated on a scale of 1–14, with 7 being a neutral solution. A pH of less than 7 indicates that the solution is acid, a reading greater than 7 that the solution is alkaline.

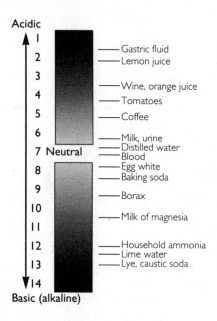

*The pH scale*

The pH of the body has to be maintained within a narrow range. The range for the blood is 7.35–7.45 – this is slightly alkaline. A pH below 6.8 and above 7.8 is regarded as harmful for the cells.

Acids are substances that release hydrogen ions in a solution; bases are substances that accept hydrogen ions. When an acid combines with a base their distinctive properties are neutralised and water and a salt are formed. This neutralisation reaction contributes to the maintenance of the pH of the body fluids.

A buffer is a compound that modifies the effect of an acid or alkali. It is added to a solution so that the pH alters only slightly. The base sodium bicarbonate acts as a buffer.

If we add sodium bicarbonate to an acid, the bicarbonate ions will combine with the free hydrogen ions to counteract the acidity. This reaction forms the basis of how antacids work to relieve excess acidity in the stomach which is felt as indigestion.

Acids can be described as strong or weak depending on the rate at which they release hydrogen ions in solution. A strong acid releases hydrogen ions easily in solution, a weak acid releases them slowly. Hydrochloric acid in the stomach is an example of a strong acid. When placed in water it shows a high concentration of hydrogen ions. Hydrochloric acid helps to prevent micro-organisms that might cause infection if they survived in the stomach. Carbonic acid formed by carbon dioxide and water is a weak acid. This acid can be found in fizzy drinks and its weakness is confirmed by the fact that it is harmless to drink.

**Care point** ▶ In certain circumstances, a person may require feeding via a tube in the stomach so that a balanced diet is given. The position of the tube is checked by obtaining a sample from the stomach content which is tested with litmus paper. If the results are acid they confirm that the tube is in the stomach and the feed can be given safely.

Buffers can combine with either an acid or an alkali to prevent excessive changes in pH. They convert a strong acid or a strong base to a weaker one, reducing the impact of the change in pH. Buffering is only temporary, however, as hydrogen ions will still need to be eliminated or retained by the body as appropriate to its needs. For example if there is an excess of hydrogen ions in the body, carbonic acid dissociates or separates to form carbon dioxide and water. The carbon dioxide will then be exhaled from the lungs and the water excreted by the kidneys.

## Breathing

Buffers work in pairs and there are several pairs in the body which complement the activities of the lungs and kidneys. The lungs regulate the amount of carbon dioxide present in the blood by removing its excess. When we breathe out, 50–75 per cent of excess carbon dioxide can be removed via this route. The respiratory centre in the brain that controls our breathing is sensitive to the concentration of hydrogen ions in body fluids and also to excess carbon dioxide. When the body fluids are too acid or there is an excess of carbon dioxide, the centre increases the rate at which we breathe, eliminating the carbon dioxide. The reduction in carbon dioxide content also affects the amount of carbonic acid that can be produced; in this way the overall acid content of the body is kept in balance.

## The effect of diet on acidity

The production of hydrogen ions varies depending on our diet, level of exercise or disease processes. This means that excretion must be regulated if a constant range of pH is to be maintained. An individual consuming a normal balanced diet has to excrete approximately 60 minimoles of hydrogen ions daily to maintain a constant range of pH in body fluids.

A diet that contains meat produces more hydrogen ions than a diet that is mainly vegetable. Vegetarians therefore produce less acid in their bodies than meat eaters.

A high level of exercise or the presence of disease processes increases the demand for energy and encourages the breakdown of stored foods, increasing the level of carbon dioxide in the blood. Some of this carbon dioxide will be exhaled while some is converted into carbonic acid.

## Acidosis and alkalosis

If breathing is inefficient, perhaps due to a lung disease such as **asthma**, the pH level will decline as carbon dioxide is retained in the body. This retention can lead to **aci-**

**dosis**, a state in which there is too much acid in the body and the pH level of the blood is therefore less than 7.35. The body compensates to restore the normal pH range by eliminating hydrogen ions by the kidneys if the lungs are not working efficiently. The pH of urine is normally 6 but will decrease in these circumstances.

If the kidneys are unable to excrete sufficient hydrogen ions, the lungs will respond by increasing the rate and depth of breaths taken, to increase the loss of carbon dioxide from the body and the subsequent carbonic acid that this would form.

A rise in pH results in **alkalosis**. This can occur if someone over-breathes from excitement or hysteria and exhales or removes a large amount of carbon dioxide from the body. In this case the elimination of carbon dioxide does not match its production. This suggests that there is too much alkali or base in the body and the pH will be more than 7.45.

The kidneys are able to excrete or retain hydrogen ions depending on the body's needs. They act at a slower rate than the lungs but are able to neutralise all excess acids or alkalis that enter the body fluids. The cells of the tubules found in the kidneys are sensitive to the pH changes in the blood. If the pH increases, the kidneys are able to remove more hydrogen ions by their formation and excretion of ammonia.

*Care point*

> Kidney functions decline with age, and the pH balance in a young adult can be restored more quickly than in an older person. The difference can be between a matter of hours or days and is worth considering if, as a carer, you are exposed to an older person who may be suffering from diabetes mellitus and may become acidotic. If the body is unable to correct the imbalance, medical treatment will be required.

## Activity 2.4

Demonstrate the range of pH in a healthy person: obtain urine samples once a day for three days from two people who are eating meat as part of their diet. Note the colour of the urine samples and test the pH with litmus paper as soon as the samples have been collected.

Obtain urine samples once a day for three days from two people who exclude meat from their diet. Note the colour of urine samples and test the pH with litmus paper as soon as possible after the samples have been collected.

Compare your readings and make comments on them.

## Twenty questions

1  Which two hormones control the loss of water and sodium in the urine?

2  Name the functional unit of the kidney.

3  Define dehydration.

4  Name the fluid compartments of the body.

5  Define fluid or water balance.

6  List the routes by which fluid is lost from the body.

**7** What are electrolytes?

**8** Define oedema.

**9** List the ways in which heat is produced in the body.

**10** What is the range of normal body temperature?

**11** List the ways in which heat is lost from the body.

**12** Define radiation, conduction and convection.

**13** What causes heat to be lost by sweating?

**14** A substance that accepts hydrogen ions is called _____

**15** A substance that releases hydrogen ions is called _____

**16** Urine contains excess hydrogen ions excreted by the kidneys and is therefore _____

**17** What is the normal pH of the blood?

**18** What is a buffer?

**19** List three factors that influence the amount of hydrogen ions produced in the body.

**20** Name two ways that acid is excreted from the body.

## Quick concepts

| | |
|---|---|
| **Acid** | A substance that accepts hydrogen ions in solution |
| **Acidosis** | A condition when in which the level of acids in the body fluids is too high |
| **Aldosterone** | A hormone released by the adrenal glands which acts on the kidney to regulate sodium and water balance |
| **Alkalosis** | A condition in which the level of alkalis in the body is too high |
| **Antidiuretic hormone** | A hormone produced by the pituitary gland that influences the concentration of urine |
| **Asthma** | A condition characterised by spasm of the bronchial tubes which results in breathing difficulties |
| **Base** | A substance that accepts hydrogen ions in a solution and releases hydroxy ions |
| **Buffer** | A substance that stabilises the pH of a solution |
| **Cell membrane** | The layer surrounding the cell |
| **Conduction** | The transfer of heat from a region of high to low temperature |
| **Convection** | Transfer of heat through a liquid or gas by movement of the heated portions |
| **Dehydration** | Excess loss of water in the body tissues |
| **Diabetes mellitus** | A disorder of carbohydrate metabolism due to lack of the hormone insulin |

| | |
|---|---|
| **Diarrhoea** | Passing of abnormally soft faeces |
| **Diffusion** | Mixing of a solution or gas with another by the movement of their particles |
| **Diuretics** | Drugs that increase the volume of urine passed |
| **Electrolytes** | Substances that dissociate in water |
| **Enzymes** | Proteins that speed up chemical reactions in the body without changing themselves in the reaction |
| **Evaporation** | Removal of water from a surface by the formation of vapour |
| **Extracellular fluid** | Fluid outside the cells |
| **Gastrointestinal tract** | The long tube that extends from the mouth to the anus, through which food passes |
| **Glomerular nephritis** | Inflammation of the kidney, usually due to an allergic response |
| **Homeostasis** | The maintenance of a constant internal environment in the body despite variations in external conditions |
| **Intracellular fluid** | The fluid medium inside the cells |
| **Liver** | The largest gland in the body found in the upper right of the abdomen |
| **Lymph** | Fluid found in the lymphatic vessels |
| **Metabolism** | Physical and chemical breakdown of food for use by the body |
| **Nephrons** | Functional units of the kidney |
| **Oedema** | Excess accumulation of water in the tissues |
| **Osmosis** | The passage of water from an area of low to higher concentration of solute |
| **pH** | The measure of acidity and alkalinity |
| **Radiation** | The spread of heat rays in the environment |
| **Stroke** | A condition in which one side of the body becomes weak due to diminished blood supply to the part of the brain that controls it |
| **Urea** | The end product of protein metabolism |

# 3 Coping mechanisms in the human body

### What is covered in this chapter

- Tissue damage
- Micro-organisms and infection
- Infectious diseases
- The immune system
- Vaccination
- Antibiotics
- The healing process

## Introduction

Every day our body defends us from bacteria and copes with damage to its tissues. If we cut ourselves in the garden we do not rush to see the doctor to get treatment – unless the cut is a large one. We may not even go indoors to wash it and yet the body manages to get rid of any potential **infection** and to heal the tissues with the minimum of scarring. When we have an operation it is the body, not modern medicine, that heals the surgeon's cut.

This chapter will provide you with knowledge and understanding about the disease process. You will learn how infection and tissue damage affect the body as well as how the body fights these processes and how healing occurs.

It is important that we understand how bacteria may enter the body and how, when they do, the body defends itself. You will learn how infection may be reduced in a hospital ward by, for example, such simple procedures as correct hand washing.

Sometimes medicines are used to encourage immunity, as in vaccinations, or to kill bacteria, as in antibiotics. You may be able to think of examples in your own life when both these methods have been put to good use. Such uses will also be discussed in this chapter.

## Tissue damage

By the time you have worked through this section you should be able to know:
- how the body's tissues may be damaged
- what the body's response is to this damage
- whether the body responds differently to infection compared to physical **trauma.**

### Inflammation

**Inflammation** is the body's local response to any injury which causes tissue damage.

The inflammatory response is one that most of us can recognise. There are four important signs:

- redness
- heat
- swelling
- pain.

There may be loss of function of the part involved due to pain on movement. The inflammatory response is the same whatever the cause of the tissue damage.

**Activity 3.1**

You can demonstrate inflammation yourself. Run the end of a blunt implement such as a match with reasonable pressure along your forearm. Observe your arm 30 seconds later. You will see that there is already a thin red line appearing. If not, you have probably been too gentle with yourself! Observe your arm again in two minutes. What is the change now? Write it down. We will discuss the reasons for this change.

You have actually just damaged the cells in your arm and inflammation occurs as a prelude to healing when tissue is damaged. However, excessive inflammation can impair healing because some of the chemicals concerned can be dangerous to the body.

### The inflammatory response

Why is the inflamed area red? Why is it hot? See if you can answer these questions before you read on.

The redness and heat mean that there is increased blood supply to the area. This brings with it more white blood cells which you will learn are very important in defence against infection and removal of dead tissue.

### Causes of inflammation

Anything that causes damage to the tissues will cause inflammation. The causes might be physical or chemical, an allergic reaction or due to living causes.

### Physical causes

- **Trauma** or physical injury: this could result in a cut, bruise or perhaps broken bone. The trauma may occur accidentally, for example by falling, or might be the result of an incident such as an assault .
- Radiation: this includes ultra violet light and you may well have experienced this form of inflammation as sunburn! The skin shows all the signs of inflammation. Patients receiving radiotherapy experience an inflammatory reaction to the treatment, which will be seen as redness of the skin.
- Intense temperatures: dry heat results in a burn; wet heat, such as boiling water, results in a scald; extreme cold may lead to frostbite.

### Chemical causes

Many chemicals cause an inflammatory response on the skin. An example would be strong acids or alkalis. If you have ever spilled acid on your hand you will have seen the immediate redness that appears on the skin. This is an inflammatory response.

### Allergic reactions

**Allergic** reactions are examples of inflammation occurring inappropriately. When we are allergic to something our body produces chemicals which give the inflammatory response. A hay fever sufferer, for example may be allergic to pollen; the chemicals produced by the body cause redness, swelling of the eyes and nasal mucosa. When mucous membranes become inflamed they overproduce mucus. A person with bad hay fever shows evidence of this with watering eyes and running nose.

The chemical responsible for this action is called histamine. The drugs taken to prevent this chemical working are called anti-histamines.

There are different types of allergies and some, such as penicillin allergy, can be extremely serious and become more pronounced each time the allergen (the chemical which produces the response) is met.

**Care point**

It is important that those in the medical profession check with a client when they are starting a course of penicillin that the client is not allergic to this drug.

### Living causes

Living causes include tiny, one-celled creatures such as bacteria and viruses as well as fungi and protozoa. These are micro-organisms, so called because they are very small and only visible under a microscope. Micro-organisms that cause disease are called **pathogens**.

This type of inflammation is said to be due to infection, which means invasion by micro-organisms and their multiplication in the tissues. In caring for clients it is important for carers to protect the patient from infection whenever possible.

The activity which follows introduces the subject of hospital-acquired infection. This topic is discussed more fully on page 43.

**Activity 3.2**

Write down the possible sources of infection for the patient in hospital. Alongside these see if you can think how the carer may help to prevent this infection.
Now think of the client in their own home and decide whether you think there is greater or lesser risk of infection here.

### Outcomes of inflammation

#### Resolution

Inflammation is a necessary prelude to healing but there may be other outcomes. Imagine you have a nice little inflamed area on your chin! Could be the beginnings of a nasty pimple! Can you think of two different outcomes?

The ideal outcome is that the inflammation subsides and the red area disappears. This would mean that the inflammatory response had effectively dealt with the cause of trauma, in this case bacteria.

When the inflammatory response is effective and tissue returns to normality without scarring, this is called resolution. Resolution occurs in:

• aseptic inflammation (no infection present), such as sunburn, for example; you may be red in the evening following exposure to the sun, but by next morning the tissues are repaired and the inflammation has gone
• when the power of the bacteria in an infection is low, and natural resistance is high. When resolution occurs:
• the body is in control
• swelling subsides

- redness disappears
- function returns.

As healing occurs scar tissue is formed.

### Suppuration

The alternative outcome is **suppuration**, the formation of pus. Pus is a thick yellow or green liquid containing dead white blood cells, living and dead bacteria and dead body cells. Once pus has formed it has to be eliminated before healing can occur. If pus forms in a confined space, this is an abscess.

### Chronic inflammation

Inflammation is chronic when it persists over a period of time and resolution is prevented, for example chronic leg ulcers, which take a very long time to heal. Leg ulcers are partly due to poor circulation, which is fairly common in elderly people. They are also associated with certain disease processes, for example diabetes mellitus.

## Activity 3.3

### Terminology

When an area of the body becomes inflamed it is given the suffix -itis; for example inflammation of the coverings of the brain, meninges, is meningitis.
Can you work out the terms for inflammation of the following:

- oesophagus
- colon
- larynx
- pharynx?

The answers will be found at the end of the chapter on page 55.

# Micro-organisms and infection

## Viruses

Viruses are the smallest of all micro-organisms and cannot be seen with a basic microscope. They actually live inside the body cells and reproduce there. This makes them much more difficult to kill. Can you think why?

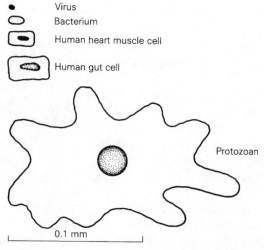

*The relative sizes of micro-organisms*

Any drug used to kill a virus is also likely to kill our cells. There are very few drug that we can use to eliminate viruses, which is why such diseases as AIDS are so diffi cult to treat. The AIDS virus lives inside one type of white cell in the blood and pre vents the cell combating infection. An AIDS sufferer may thus die from an infection that a person without the virus would easily resist.

Not all viruses are as dangerous as the HIV virus which causes AIDS. The com mon cold is a viral illness that most of us manage to take in our stride. However, ever mild illnesses like this can present dangers to the very old  and very young whose immune systems may not be functioning to their full capacity.

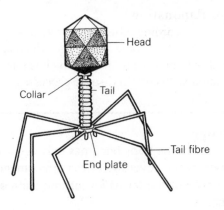

*A diagrammatic representation of one type of virus*

Many common childhood illnesses are due to viruses. Chickenpox, for example is caused by one form of the Herpes virus, herpes zoster, which can lie dormant in the body and reactivate as shingles. Another form of herpes causes cold sores. This is her pes simplex. It, too, can lie dormant and recur when a person is tired or stressed.

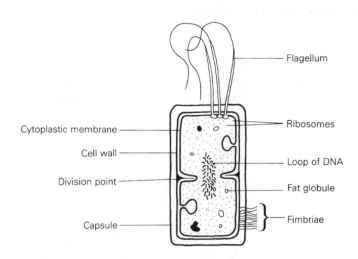

*A typical bacterium*

## Bacteria

Bacteria are the commonest micro-organisms to cause infection in the human body They are minute organisms made from only one cell. Three hundred of them could be placed end to end across a pin head, so you cannot see them with the naked eye

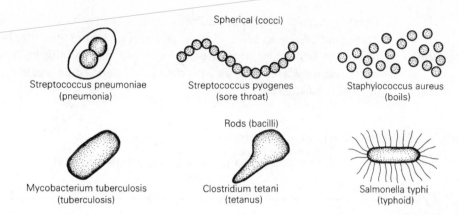

Spherical (cocci)

Streptococcus pneumoniae
(pneumonia)

Streptococcus pyogenes
(sore throat)

Staphylococcus aureus
(boils)

Rods (bacilli)

Mycobacterium tuberculosis
(tuberculosis)

Clostridium tetani
(tetanus)

Salmonella typhi
(typhoid)

*Examples of bacteria*

They come in different shapes. Some are round, some are in chains and some are rod-shaped.

Some bacteria are pathogenic and cause disease in man. They do so by destroying healthy tissues for their own survival, often producing poisons (toxins) in the process. However, not all bacteria are harmful. Some of them are useful to man:

- the bacteria which decompose and break down dead plant and animal matter; imagine what would happen if all the living waste over the ages did not rot. Think of walking in the forest with all the leaves of many years to wade through! The same bacterial mechanisms also decompose sewage
- the bacteria which are important in the food industry, for example those which turn cream into cheese and help to make yoghurt
- bacteria which we have in our intestines that help to provide the vitamins we do not obtain in our diet
- bacteria from which antibiotics are obtained.

Although these bacteria are helpful, along with some other parasites including viruses, fungi and protozoa, other bacteria may cause many forms of disease and are responsible for many deaths.

# Infectious diseases

Infectious diseases cause less than two per cent of deaths in the western world but are still responsible for more visits to the local doctor than any other single cause. In developing countries they are still responsible for 70–80 per cent of deaths.

## Activity 3.4

Why do infectious diseases kill more people in the developing countries?

Go to your local library, choose a developing country and see if you can find out what percentage of people die due to infections. Look also for the explanation of this high death toll. Oxfam may be able to supply you with useful information in this area.

It is not just due to lack of medical facilities that people die, but also because of malnutrition, poor sanitation, overcrowding, contaminated food and water and poor vaccination programmes. People's resistance to disease is lowered because their natural defences are lowered.

**Care point**

Certain patients in hospital and the community may have their defences lowered. This could be due to other chronic sickness or loss of appetite, leading to malnutrition. All bodily functions lose efficiency with age and this includes the ability to resist disease. Care workers with the elderly need to be particularly careful not to introduce infection.

## Portals of entry for micro-organisms

How do harmful bacteria and other invaders enter the body?

**Activity 3.5**

Write down the infections that you and your family have had in the past year. See if you can work out the route of entry for the micro-organism; write this down before you read further.

| Possible routes of entry | Possible resulting infections |
|---|---|
| Respiratory tract | Common cold |
| | Tuberculosis |
| Alimentary tract (through the mouth and into the gut) | Salmonella |
| Break in the skin or mucous membranes | Wound infection |
| | Tetanus |
| Bloodstream | Malaria |
| | Hepatitis B |

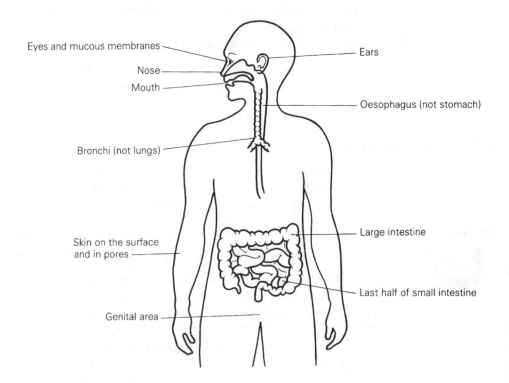

*Portals of entry for micro-organisms*

**Care point**

When caring for the sick it is important that infection is not transferred from one person to another (cross infection). One way to help prevent this is by always washing the hands after caring for one client, before moving to the next.

## Hospital-acquired infection

Hospitals can be a source of infections that a client would have been safe from at home. You thought about this in Activity 3.2 on page 38 and we now give some of the reasons why hospitals are often more at risk from micro-organisms than the client's own home.

- A large number of people are brought together, each with their own population of micro-organisms.
- The hospital has its own population of micro-organisms; these tend to be more both virulent and resistant to many antibiotics.
- Some treatments given in hospital render the patient more susceptible to infection; for example radiotherapy may interfere with the body's ability to make white blood cells.

Hospital-acquired infections tend to fall into three categories:

- wound infections
- chest infections
- urinary tract infections.

In all cases the carer can help to prevent infection by:

- hand washing between caring for different patients; this reduces the risk of cross-infection from one client to another

Spread of infection from nose, throat, skin, intestines
Poor technique and discipline of staff:

- dirty apron
- failure to wash hands
- long hair, nails
- touching sterile dressings, peking under dressings

The patient's own organisms: spreading infection from nose/gut to wound via fingers

Other patients sit on beds, share food, magazines, etc.

**Airborne particles** carry bacteria

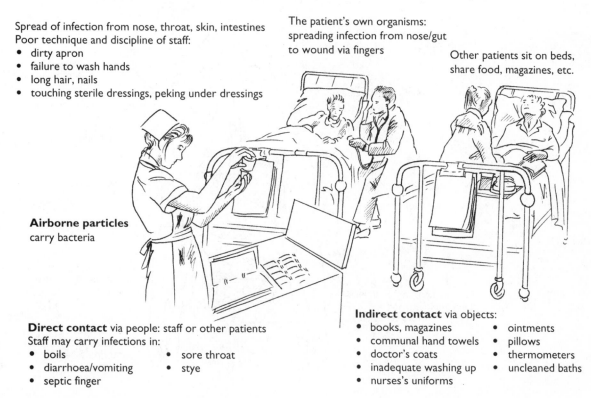

**Direct contact** via people: staff or other patients
Staff may carry infections in:

- boils
- diarrhoea/vomiting
- septic finger
- sore throat
- stye

**Indirect contact** via objects:

- books, magazines
- communal hand towels
- doctor's coats
- inadequate washing up
- nurses's uniforms
- ointments
- pillows
- thermometers
- uncleaned baths

*Common sources of infection in a hospital*

- the use of gloves when dealing with any body fluids
- the use of aseptic technique when attending to wounds; this means using a procedure to maintain sterility – the use of sterile gloves, for example – and each hospital has its own procedure documented for nurses to follow. Most clean wounds that become infected do so on the wards.

# The immune system

The immune system is the body's defence system against disease and helps to protect us from everything from a common cold to cancer. The system is still not entirely understood and research in this field is continually progressing.

Some parts of our immune system are present at birth. These parts are called the **innate immune system**. They use the same defence against all types of infection. In other words they are non-specific. They would respond in exactly the same way whether you had whooping cough or measles.

Other parts of the immune system are **adaptive** and make specific antibodies to each disease we meet. These antibodies defend us against that disease but not against any other. The antibodies against whooping cough, for example, will not protect against measles.

## The innate immune system

The innate (inborn) immune system is made up of several different forms of protection which can be placed in two categories:
- physical and chemical barriers to infection
- white blood cells that engulf bacteria.

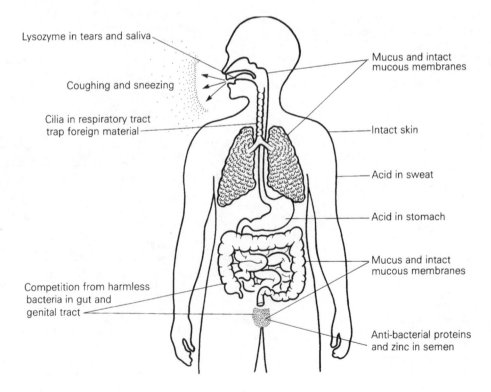

Lysozyme in tears and saliva

Coughing and sneezing

Cilia in respiratory tract trap foreign material

Competition from harmless bacteria in gut and genital tract

Mucus and intact mucous membranes

Intact skin

Acid in sweat

Acid in stomach

Mucus and intact mucous membranes

Anti-bacterial proteins and zinc in semen

*The physical, chemical and mechanical barriers to infection*

### Physical and chemical barriers
- The skin: this is the body's first line of defence. As long as it is unbroken, most pathogens (see page 38) cannot penetrate it. When this barrier is broken, as in bad burns, there is real danger of infection.
- Mucous membranes: they line the body tracts, for example the gut.
- Sweat: an acid secretion that inhibits bacterial growth.
- Acid (in the stomach): it destroys many of the micro-organisms that are present in the food we eat.
- Lysozyme: this is an enzyme present in tears, milk, saliva and other secretions. It digests bacterial cell walls.
- Cilia are little hairs that line the respiratory tract and trap bacteria. They beat to move bacteria towards the exterior.
- Coughing and sneezing effectively expel micro-organisms trapped in the mucus.

Coughs and sneezes also expel micro-organisms into the atmosphere. 'Coughs and sneezes spread diseases': nothing could be more true!

### White blood cells
The process by which white blood cells engulf bacteria is called **phagocytosis** and is described on page 47.

## Blood

Blood is a fluid contained within a closed system of vessels: the arteries, veins and capillaries through which it is made to circulate by the pumping action of the heart. Blood consists of a yellow liquid (plasma), large numbers of cells (corpuscles), and cell fragments (platelets).

Plasma contains blood proteins, inorganic salts, food substances, waste materials, enzymes, hormones, antimicrobial substances and vitamins. Plasma makes up 55 per cent of blood and cells make up approximately 45 per cent.

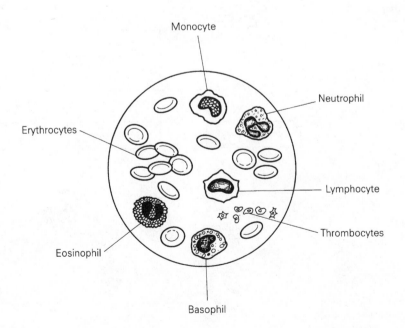

*The types of cell found in the blood*

Blood acts as a transport system around the body. It transports oxygen and nutrients to the cells so that they have energy to function. It transports carbon dioxide and other waste products away from the cells to be eliminated. Exchanges between plasma and tissue fluid take place through the thin walls of the capillaries.

There are three types of cell found in the blood:

- red cells (erythrocytes), which carry oxygen to the tissues. These are biconcave discs without a nucleus and only live about 120 days. Their main function is to transport oxygen attached to a pigment called haemoglobin which gives the erythrocyte its red colour. If there is too little haemoglobin in the body, the person is anaemic. To make haemoglobin, the body needs iron
- platelets, which take part in the clotting process. These are very small cells which are concerned with the arrest of bleeding. They stick together and form a 'platelet plug' when we cut ourselves. Clotting follows
- white cells (leucocytes). There are several different types of white cell. They are all concerned with fighting disease and are made in the bone marrow. Leukaemia occurs when white cells overproduce and are immature.

**Care point**

A person with leukaemia has immature white cells that cannot function. This means that the person is very susceptible to disease as they do not have the ability to fight off infections. When caring for such people extra precautions are taken to reduce the risk of infection. These might include nursing the client in a single room and not allowing those with infections such as colds to visit.

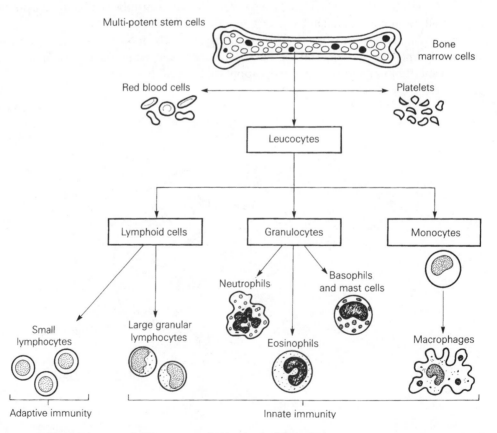

*The development of different types of white blood cell from the bone marrow*

There are three main types of white cell in the blood:
- lymphocytes: the smallest white cells, which make antibodies to disease. We will be discussing these below as part of the adaptive immune system. 5 per cent of lymphocytes are larger than the rest and form part of the innate system. They produce chemicals to kill viruses.
- neutrophils: these can engulf bacteria. They are the white cells that are first attracted to an area of inflammation. They will then engulf both bacteria and dead tissue. By so doing they help in the healing process.
- monocytes: these are more concerned with chronic infection and inflammation. They live longer and can enter the tissues to fight infection there. When in the tissues they become larger and are called macrophages.

When there is infection in the body, the number of white cells in the blood increases. A doctor may take a sample of blood and send it to a laboratory for a white cell count. The normal number of white cells is between five and nine million per millilitre of blood.

### Phagocytosis

Phagocytosis is a process used by simple organisms, such as amoeba (see Chapter 1), to engulf food particles. The amoeba can change shape, and when it approaches a food particle extends out projections called pseudopodia, with which it completely surrounds the particle.

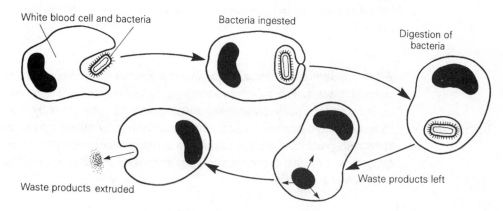

*Phagocytosis of a bacteria by a white blood cell*

Some scientists think that the white blood cell is related to the amoeba. It engulfs bacteria and dead tissue in exactly the same manner, as shown in the illustration above. When the blood cell has completely enclosed the bacteria in a membrane lined cavity, it releases deadly enzymes which digest the bacteria and kill it. Any indigestible remains, now harmless, are expelled from the white cell which is then free to catch other bacteria and repeat the process. Some bacteria have learned to resist this chemical breakdown by the white cell. One such example is the tubercle bacillus which causes tuberculosis. This bacteria can actually live inside the phagocyte.

There may also be problems if the white cell engulfs indigestible material such as, for example, coal dust in the lungs. The white cell produces more and more chemicals to try to destroy the dust and eventually dies, releasing the destructive chemicals into the lung tissue. This is the cause of pneumoconiosis, a type of lung damage that occurs in coal miners and can lead to a severe form of chronic bronchitis.

### Killer cells

Killer cells are a type of large lymphocyte. They are white blood cells that can kill viruses. They cannot engulf like the neutrophils but release chemicals such as interferon, which has been tried as a cure for cancer. These chemicals protect the body against many viral infections and prevent the virus replicating. It is believed that they also provide protect against tumour growth.

## The adaptive immune system

As mentioned earlier (page 44), the adaptive immune system is specific and responds differently to different infections. It involves the white cell called the lymphocyte.

### T cells and B cells

There are two types of small lymphocyte that cannot be distinguished under the microscope. These are T cells and B cells. Both originate in the bone marrow, but T cells mature in the thymus gland in the neck. It is thought that B cells mature in the bone marrow.

The B cells make antibodies. The T cells regulate the immune response by releasing chemicals to stimulate or suppress **antibody** production. They take part in inflammation and also in cytotoxicity (cell killing). In cases of AIDS, the virus attacks the T cell and the victim cannot then make antibodies effectively; as stated previously (page 40) the patient dies from infections against which others without the virus could defend themselves.

**Care point**

AIDS is essentially a sexually transmitted disease, by either homosexual or heterosexual contacts. The other two main routes of transmission are via infected blood or from an infected mother to the uterus and her unborn baby. AIDS cannot be caught through normal contact and certainly not by talking to the patient! However, great care must be taken to protect health workers when they are in contact with blood or blood products and when handling body fluids. Gloves must be worn at these times.

**Activity 3.6**

Investigate the policy of your local hospital towards clients with AIDS. Make notes of the precautions recommended. What do you think are the psychological dangers to the client of having such policies?

### Antibodies

Anything which stimulates antibody production by the lymphocytes is called an **antigen**. Bacteria, viruses, fungi, and all foreign (for example, transplanted) cells have antigens on their surface. These antigens stimulate the body to make antibodies against them.

The illustration at the top of the next page shows a bacteria. On its surface are antigens. The antibodies are made in response to these antigens and will fit and lock onto them.

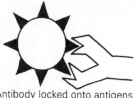

Bacteria with
antigens attached

Antibody that will
fit the antigens

Antibody locked onto antigens
(Not drawn to scale)

*Bacteria with antigens*

### Specificity of antibodies

An antibody will only combine with only one type of antigen; in other words it is specific (see page 00). This means that if you have had measles and have made antibodies to this virus, those antibodies will only protect you from measles and not against any other disease.

When an antibody has attached itself to an antigen it is called an immune complex and is much more easily attacked by the phagocytes in the body. This means that if the body make antibodies to bacteria, these will attach themselves to the antigens on the bacterial cell surface and then the phagocytes will be able to engulf and kill them.

### Auto-immune disease

It is very important that the body does not make antibodies to itself or we would destroy our own body tissues. Normally this does not happen as the body can differentiate between self and non-self. When the system does occasionally go wrong, an auto-immune disease such as rheumatoid arthritis may occur. Auto-immune diseases are not uncommon. The body makes antibodies to, and starts to destroy, its own joints causing inflammation and pain. The joints are often very swollen and painful and even the touch of bed sheets on the knees may cause pain.

### The memory of the lymphocytes

**Activity 3.7**

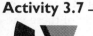

Write down three infectious diseases you have had, probably as a child, or that your children have had. Now tick those that you have had more than once.

There will usually be no ticks! The immune system remembers the micro-organism and protection is so fast that we do not become ill with the disease. It is because of this memory that our response to an infection the second time we meet it is much more effective.

The primary response occurs the first time we meet an antigen. It takes the lymphocytes several days to start to make sufficient antibodies against the bacteria or virus. If you have had the disease before, the secondary response occurs and the immune system remembers the disease and makes the antibodies very quickly. The disease therefore tends to spread less rapidly in the body during the secondary response stage than it would in the primary response stage.

**Activity 3.8**

Look at the two graphs at the top of the next page. The left-hand graph shows a primary response to infection and the right-hand a secondary response. Write down three differences between the two responses shown. This principle is used in vaccination, which is discussed in the next section.

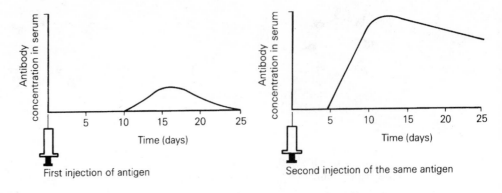

First injection of antigen          Second injection of the same antigen

## Vaccination

Edward Jenner was the first person to use **vaccination**, in 1796. An injection of dead or weakened micro-organisms is given which is sufficient to stimulate the immune response but insufficient actually to produce the disease. This is the primary response. When the person comes into contact with the disease at a later date the immune system remembers and quickly produces sufficient antibodies to prevent illness .A secondary response to the infection has occurred.

Vaccination is one form of immunisation, which is the production of immunity by artificial means. There are two possible types of immunity that may be given: active or passive.

## Active immunity

Vaccination can provide **active immunity**. The body has to make its own antibodies to the disease. This means that the lymphocytes will have a memory for the antigen and that protection will be long-lasting. Children are now vaccinated against the commoner infectious diseases of childhood. A table showing the timing of these vaccinations is shown below.

### Immunisation schedules

| Vaccine | Age | Notes |
|---|---|---|
| Diphtheria, tetanus, pertussis, haemophilus, influenzae (Hib), polio | | Primary course |
| 1st dose | 2 months | |
| 2nd dose | 3 months | |
| 3rd dose | 4 months | |
| Measles/mumps/rubella (MMR) | 12–15 months | Can be given at any age over 12 months |
| Booster D/T and polio, MMR (if not previously given) | 3–5 years | |
| Rubella | 10–14 years | Girls only |
| BCG | 10–14 years or infancy | Intervals of 3 weeks between BCG and rubella |
| Booster tetanus and polio | 15–19 years | |

## Passive immunity

**Passive immunity** is a temporary measure and involves the administration of the actual antibodies to the disease in the form of gamma globulin. If, for example, someone is bitten by a dog in a country where rabies is still a danger, they are given the antibodies to rabies which offer a temporary but immediate protection. It is possible to protect against many diseases in this manner. The donated antibodies are foreign to the body and are destroyed. This explains why this type of immunity is short-lived. No permanent protection results.

### Immune globulin

**Immune globulin** is a sterile solution containing many of the antibodies found in an adult's blood. It is prepared from plasma pooled from the venous blood of more than 1000 individuals. It is given to those who have an immunodeficiency disorder, and is also used to give passive immunity to those exposed to an infection.

### Risks in pooling plasma

Can you see any possible dangers in the pooling of plasma from many individuals?

It may be possible that some of the donors have infections in their blood such as hepatitis or HIV. Manufacturers have to test donated plasma to ensure that antigens to these two diseases are not present. As an extra precaution, since April 1985, the manufacturing process includes highly effective steps to remove or inactivate the HIV virus.

# Antibiotics

Most of the time our immune response enables our white blood cells to kill and consume microscopic organisms. In some instances, however, the body needs some assistance to help it to control infection. Ever since the discovery that bacteria caused infection, man has been trying to find a way of eliminating these tiny organisms without causing damage to himself. Antibiotics are substances produced by, or derived from micro-organisms. They either kill or inhibit the growth of bacteria, fungi or viruses.

Antibiotic drugs have revolutionised the treatment of infections and diseases that used to cause many deaths. Meningitis, for example can now be cured, although it is necessary to detect the disease at an early stage and commence antibiotic therapy, as some forms of meningitis can still be lethal.

The discovery of antibiotics does not mean that the battle against micro-organisms is over. Many bacteria have become resistant to certain antibiotics which now no longer kill them.

## How do antibiotics work?

Antibiotics work by destroying the outer membrane of the bacteria or stop the bacteria reproducing. It is essential that the antibiotic does not destroy the cells of the host (i.e. man). There are still very few antibiotics that work against viruses. This is because the virus actually lives inside the host cell. Any drug that destroys the virus is likely to destroy the host cell as well.

## Resistance

Resistance occurs when the bacteria alter their chemical structure so that the antibiotic no longer kills them. Certain strains of bacteria, for example the staphylococcus, have become quite adept at this and have necessitated the constant search for new drugs. Many hospitals have a problem with a strain of staphylococcus that is multi-resistant. This bacteria has become resistant to many antibiotics and may infect wounds. It can be carried in the throats or on the skin of staff who do not know they are harbouring the bacterium.

## Penicillin

Penicillin was discovered by Alexander Fleming in 1928. It is still one of the most popular antibiotics today due to its effectiveness, safety and low cost. Scientists have now made many different forms of penicillins that differ slightly in their chemical structure and so can attack a wider variety of bacteria. Examples you may have heard of, or actually taken yourself are ampicillin, amoxycillin and flucloxacillin.

### Routes of administration

Most antibiotics can be given orally (by mouth) but if a person is very ill, the doctor may choose to give the drug intravenously (directly into the bloodstream).

*Care point* ▶ If we are caring for someone receiving antibiotics it is most important that we advise them to finish the course, even if they are already feeling better. Incomplete courses allow some bacteria to survive and to become resistant to the drug. Antibiotics are usually prescribed for periods of five days or one week.

## Viral infections

We have already mentioned that viruses are very difficult to kill (page 51) and ordinary antibiotics such as penicillin will have no effect on a viral disease. That is why it is of no benefit to receive an antibiotic for a common cold. It will still last for exactly the same length of time.

## Natural resistance

Even when antibiotics are used, it must be remembered that the natural resistance of the body still plays an important part in combating disease. Man, as a species, survived for many thousands of years before the advent of antibiotics. Healing and the immune response are totally natural processes. They are completely automatic and usually occur without medical aid. They are able to start and stop as required. Medicine, especially surgery, may need them more than they need medicine!

## The healing process

If we suffer a small scratch or cut in the kitchen the body will effectively stop the bleeding and heal the cut. After a few days the scab will fall off and within about two weeks all sign of injury will have gone. Any micro-organisms that were contaminating the cut will have been disposed of by the body's defences.

Healing is the body's replacement of destroyed tissue by living tissue and takes place in three overlapping phases:
- inflammation
- reconstruction
- maturation.

Inflammation as a prelude to healing has already been discussed (pages 36–7).

# Reconstruction

The emphasis is now on repair and large numbers of body cells called fibroblasts are busy producing new tissue. When the wound edges are opposed repair can take place immediately. This is the case in small cuts and after surgery when sutures are holding the wound together.

# Maturation

Maturation is the period of remodelling of scar tissue. It may continue for many months if the wound is large.

## Activity 3.9

Think back to the last time you were ill with an infection. Make a list of the factors you feel may have aided your recovery. Check your list with the one which follows.

## Factors that influence recovery

### Rest
When we have an infection it can affect the whole body. Even if the infection is localised to one area, for example an abscess, if it is severe it will also have systemic effects (i.e. affect the whole body). The treatment for a severe infection usually includes rest, and if the infection is severe enough, the body may enforce rest on the patient, who feels too weak to go about normal activities.

### Diet
Diet can affect recovery; if we have been eating a well-balanced diet with all the necessary vitamins and minerals, we are better able to fight any infection.

### Rise in body temperature
An infection often causes a rise in body temperature (**pyrexia**). Scientists still do not understand how this aids recovery.

### Healthy immune system
A healthy immune system, as we have seen above, will be essential in any recovery. Those whose immune systems are unable to cope may die from infections that healthy people can easily resist.

### Freedom from other disease
If there is another underlying disease present, the body will find it more difficult to rid itself of infection; for example, following a stroke or after an operation, the resistance to infection will be lower and there is more danger of, say, chest infections turning into pneumonia.

### Age
Age is an important factor in response to infection; the very young and the very old are less able to respond adequately.

Not all wounds are as straight forward as a simple clean cut; you may have seen leg ulcers or pressure sores where healing is often difficult and delayed. One reason for this may be the age of the client – healing is just one of the body's processes that become less efficient as the body grows older.

**Care point** ▷ The elderly may not respond to an infection with an increase in temperature, so they may be more seriously ill than their signs might indicate. Even with quite severe infections, temperature may be normal. Less sensitivity to pain can add to the dangers.

## Factors that delay healing

There are several factors which can delay the healing process:
- old age
- the presence of a generalised infection
- poor nutritional status
- a weak immune system
- poor blood supply to the wound
- infection in the wound
- difficult position of the wound
- the wound is very deep
- the presence of other disease, for example cancer, anaemia, diabetes.

To encourage fast healing we must try to ensure that we fulfil as many of the criteria needed for healing as possible. This includes keeping the wound clean and free from infection and ensuring that the client has a diet with the necessary vitamins and protein.

> **Case study**
> Mrs Budd is an elderly diabetic with a leg ulcer. She is having the ulcer dressed twice a week and feels she is taking all the advice the nurse gives. However, the ulcer seems no nearer to healing than it was three months ago. Mrs Budd is now becoming depressed and is no longer preparing balanced meals. Some of the factors that delay healing are present in her case: she is elderly, not eating well and has diabetes. Her leg ulcer is probably also deep. She will need advice from the carer, not just on the healing of her ulcer but also on the best foods to eat.

## Twenty questions

1 What are the four signs of inflammation?

2 Name four causes of inflammation.

3 Which naturally occurring chemical in the body is responsible for an allergic response such as hay fever?

4 What is suppuration?

5 What are the smallest micro-organisms called?

6 Name four routes of entry for micro-organisms into the body.

7 Which part of the immune system is present at birth?

8 What is lysozyme?

9 Where are white blood cells made?

10 What is an antigen?

11  Describe how an antibody works.

12  The carer of a child asks you how vaccination works; write down your explanation.

13  What are the differences between active and passive immunity?

14  Hospital-acquired infections tend to fall into three categories; what are these

15  What is cross-infection?

16  In what ways can a carer help to prevent cross-infection occurring on a hospital ward?

17  What are the three stages of the healing process?

18  Why are viruses so difficult to kill?

19  Why are the very old and the very young in more danger from infections?

20  How is the AIDS virus transmitted?

# Quick concepts

| | |
|---|---|
| **Active immunity** | The production by the body of its own antibodies to disease following vaccination or an attack of the disease |
| **Adaptive immunity** | Specific immunity involving lymphocytes and the manufacture of antibodies |
| **Allergy** | A hypersensitivity to certain antigens called allergens |
| **Antibody** | A special protein that combines with an antigen to make it less harmful and more attractive to the phagocytes (see Phagocytosis) |
| **Antigen** | Part of an immunogen that stimulates antibody production |
| **Asepsis** | Absence of micro-organisms that cause disease |
| **Immune globulin** | A sterile solution containing most of the antibodies found in an adult's blood |
| **Immunity** | The body's ability to resist infection |
| **Immunogen** | A substance which stimulates antibody production |
| **Infection** | Invasion of the body by pathogens |
| **Inflammation** | Local response to tissue damage |
| **Innate immunity** | Part of the immune response that is present at birth and is non-specific |
| **Pathogens** | Micro-organisms that cause disease |
| **Passive immunity** | A short lived immunity given by the receipt of ready-made antibodies |
| **Phagocytosis** | The engulfing and digestion of bacteria and other foreign particles by a cell |
| **Pyrexia** | A rise above normal in body temperature |
| **Suppuration** | The production of pus |
| **Trauma** | A physical wound or injury |
| **Vaccination** | A preparation of dead or drowsy micro-organisms used to stimulate antibody production |

Answers to Activity 3.3 (page 39): Oesophagitis; Colitis; Laryngitis; Pharyngitis

# 4 Food, diet and nutrition

## What is covered in this chapter

- Factors which influence diet
- Signs of good nutrition
- A healthy diet
- The digestive system
- Specific dietary plans
- Food production
- Food hygiene

## Introduction

Excessive consumption of food by the population in Britain and other developed countries poses a major threat to health, while in the developing world, the major threats to much ill-health and premature death are starvation, under-**nutrition** and deficiencies of essential **nutrients**.

In 1991 The Committee of Medical Aspects on Food Policy (COMA) published comprehensive recommendations for nutrient consumption by the population in it report *Dietary Reference Values for Food Energy and Nutrients for the United Kingdom*. The COMA report has been accepted as government policy, and government agencies, including the Ministry of Agriculture, Fisheries and Food are obliged to put it recommendations into effect. In July 1992 the Government published *The Health of the Nation*, a national strategy for health, which sets targets for, among other topics, eating behaviour, establishing nutritional status (the state of health produced by the balance between nutritional requirement and intake) and reducing diet-related diseases. These documents set the targets for **nutrition** and health standards in the different countries of the UK for the foreseeable future.

## Factors which influence diet

Factors which influence the type or quantity if food people eat can be summarised a follows (some factors are themselves influenced by others in the list):
- availability of food
- climate
- local soil type
- storage facilities
- water supply
- transport
- culture and beliefs
- personal preferences
- health status
- economic circumstances.

The availability of food will be influenced by physical and geographical factors such as the local soil type, the climate, storage facilities, water supply and the transport network. Availabilty will also depend on what can be bought locally. Shops stock food they expect to sell, and the range of products stocked may vary in poor and affluent areas.

Cultural and personal choices influence the food we eat. We choose foods we enjoy eating. If an individual dislikes a food or avoids eating a particular food, this may be because of belief that the particular food may harm them in some way, or because of physiological intolerance, for example an allergy to cheese or other dairy products. Our early life also has an effect on our choice of food. Human beings are creatures of habit, and if a child has been brought up with certain foods in his diet, these are likely to remain in the diet.

Economic influences can have a very restricting effect on the range of foods available to a family. A balanced diet can be bought on a low income, but some foods are very expensive and people on low incomes will not buy them.

A valuable source of information about dietary habits in different socio-economic groups is *The Dietary and Nutritional Survey of British Adults* (see *Supplementary Reading*, page 73), available from most local libraries. Students interested in dietetics, the study of the practical application of nutritional science to people in various conditions of health and disease, may find it a useful reference for this unit.

## Activity 4.1

What do you consider to be the major influence on the diet of a group of 7-year-old schoolchildren in an inner city area? Why do you think this influence so important?

## Signs of good nutrition

The body of scientific knowledge governing the food requirements of humans for maintenance, growth, activity, reproduction and lactation is nutritional science. **Nutrition** concerns the food people eat and how their bodies use it. Certain nutrients in the food we eat are essential to our health and well being. Food and nutrition guides help us to plan a balanced diet according to individual need and goals. The dietician on the health care team carries the major responsibility for nutritional care of clients.

Good nutrition is essential for good health throughout life, from before birth right through old age. Food has always been one of the necessities of life. We are all aware that food relieves hunger or satisfies our appetite, but we may not be too concerned whether it supplies the body with all the components of good nutrition.

The signs of good nutrition are:
- a well developed body
- ideal weight for body composition
- good muscle development and tone
- clear and smooth skin
- bright and clear eyes
- alert facial expressions
- alert – physically and mentally
- normal appetite, digestion and elimination

- positive outlook on life
- ability to resist infection and disease.

(It must be remembered that other factors as well as diet contribute to overall health and fitness. Exercise, for example, plays an important contribution.)

# A healthy diet

A healthy diet contains proteins, carbohydrates, fibre, fats, vitamins and essential minerals. A balance of different food is required to maintain health, to help create healthier people and extend the years of normal functioning. Some of the different groups of chemicals which make up a healthy human diet are now discussed.

## Protein

Protein is the fundamental structural material of every cell in the body. It makes up the bulk of the muscle, internal organs, brain, skin and has a vital role in the regulatory substances such as enzymes, hormones and blood plasma. The primary functions of protein are to repair worn out, wasted, or damaged tissue and to build new tissue.

All protein is made up of building units or compounds known as amino acids. These are joined in unique chain sequence to form specific proteins.

Protein is found in many everyday foods, such as eggs, milk, cheese, fish and meat. In a mixed diet, animal and plant foods provide a wide variety of **nutrients**. Proteins derived from foods of animal origin – milk, eggs, fish and meat – are able to supply the essential amino acids and are known as first class or complete proteins. Proteins derived from plant sources – grains, legumes, nuts, seeds, cereals and vegetables – are relatively deficient in their content of essential amino acids, and are called second class or incomplete proteins.

## Carbohydrate

Carbohydrates occur in food such as sugars and starches and are a major source of energy (as well as of dietary fibre) in the diet. Plants build up carbohydrate through the process of photosynthesis. Animals are unable to synthesise carbohydrates (one of the main differences between plants and animals).

Carbohydrates are composed of carbon, hydrogen, and oxygen. They are classified according to the number of sugar units making up their structure:
- **monosaccharides** with one sugar unit
- **disaccharides** with two sugar units
- **polysaccharides** with many sugar units.

Monosaccharides and disaccharides are simple carbohydrates, and polysaccharides are complex carbohydrates. Monosaccharides are the simple sugars of which three are important in our diet: glucose, fructose and galactose.

### Monosaccharides
#### Glucose
Glucose is a moderately sweet sugar found in honey and glucose syrup. It also comes from the digestion of polysaccharides and disaccharides in the body. It is the primary fuel source for the cells.

#### Fructose
Fructose is found mainly in fruits and honey. The amount of fructose in fruit depends

on its degree of ripeness. As the fruit ripens, some of the stored starch turns to sugar. Fructose is the sweetest of the simple sugars. Glucose and fructose are used extensively by food manufacturers to sweeten their products.

### Galactose
Galactose comes mainly from the digestion of milk sugar, lactose, which is a **disaccharide**.

These simple sugars are absorbed from the intestine into the bloodstream and carried to the liver where they may be used for immediate energy or, if they are excess to the body's needs, they may be converted by enzymes into glycogen. Glycogen is a constant back-up energy supply. It is a means of storing carbohydrate in a form which is readily converted back to glucose for energy.

### Disaccharides
There are three disaccharides in the human diet: sucrose, lactose and maltose. Sucrose is granulated table sugar refined from sugar cane and sugar beet. Lactose is sugar in milk. Maltose does not occur naturally; it is produced by fermenting grains and is present in beer and cereals.

### Polysaccharides
Complex carbohydrates are composed of glucose molecules joined together in different ways. Polysaccharides or starches are found in grains, lentils, beans, potatoes and vegetables. The more complex carbohydrates take longer to digest into simple carbohydrates such as glucose, ready for absorption, and release energy slowly over a longer period of time.

## Fibre

Dietary fibre comes from wholemeal bread, wholegrain cereals, vegetables and fruit. Western diet has a low fibre content, which has been linked to the increased incidence of some degenerative diseases. In the United Kingdom, five million prescriptions for laxatives and purgatives are written each year as treatments for constipation. More fibre in the diet would prevent this. The increased consumption of fat and sugar has been linked to the increase in obesity. By increasing unrefined carbohydrate in a calorie-controlled diet, the food stays in the stomach longer and it prolongs the feeling of fullness after a meal; unrefined carbohydrate also takes longer to eat. The incidence of diabetes mellitus, colonic disorders and carcinoma of the colon might be reduced by increasing fibre in the diet.

Most of us need to increase our daily intake of fibre, but the intake should be increased slowly over a period of time, to prevent the abdomen becoming uncomfortable and distended. If the large bowel adapts slowly to the increased fibre over a period of a few weeks, any problems, such as the embarrassment of increased wind, are lessened.

## Fats

Fats are important in nutrition as the most compact energy source available. They play an important role in body **metabolism**. They are the richest of all natural sources of energy. One gram of fat provides about 9 kcal of energy, about twice as much as a gram of sugar or protein.

Fat in foods supplies essential diet and body tissue needs, both as an energy fuel

**59**

and a structural material. Excess fat is stored in the body as adipose tissue. Fats also form an essential part of cell membranes.

**Summary of energy values**

|  | kg/g | kcal/g |
|---|---|---|
| Protein | 17 | 4 |
| Fats | 8 | 9 |
| Carbohydrate | 17 | 4 |

# Vitamins

Vitamins are needed in small amounts for healthy growth and development. Mostly they cannot be synthesised by the body and so are required as part of a healthy diet. They may be the catalysts for some reactions required to utilise proteins, fats and carbohydrates for energy, growth and cell maintenance.

There are two major groups of vitamins: fat-soluble and water-soluble.

# Fat-soluble vitamins

Vitamins A, D, E and K are fat-soluble and stored in the body for long periods of time.

### Vitamin A

Vitamin A is found in milk, fat, butter, cod liver oil and liver. It is also manufactured by the body from beta-carotene which is found in carrots and green leafy vegetables such as cabbage. It has many roles in the body, for example strengthening the skin, the lungs and the gastro-intestinal tract against infection. It is also required for normal bone growth and development. Dry skin and night blindness (nyctalopia) are important signs of deficiency.

### Vitamin D

Vitamin D is required for mineralisation of bones and teeth and for regulation of blood calcium levels. The main sources are fish oils, liver, butter and egg yolks. Vitamin D is also synthesised in the skin by the action of ultra-violet light on the skin. In adults a deficiency leads to osteomalacia, or soft bones.

**Care point** ▷ Deficiency of vitamin D and rickets is more common in children of Asian parentage in this country, as they are often strict vegetarians and lack the necessary sunlight in Britain to manufacture this vitamin in their skin. Their carers need to be encouraged to use vitamin supplements for their children to prevent rickets.

### Vitamin E

Vitamin E is found in vegetable oils, whole grains, wheat germ, leafy vegetables, egg yolks and legumes. It is widely distributed in the diet and deficiency is unlikely. The vitamin has antioxidant properties which may help the body's immune system to function and provide some protection against cancer. This vitamin has received widespread publicity in the media and has probably been credited with some properties it does not possess. Research has shown that taking Vitamin E does not improve athletic performance or increase fertility.

## Vitamin K

Vitamin K is found in green leafy vegetables, cauliflower, soybean oil and liver. It is required for the manufacture of prothrombin, a substance needed for blood clotting to occur. Deficiency rarely occurs in health as the vitamin is also synthesised by bacteria in the large bowel.

# Water soluble vitamins

## B-vitamins

The B-vitamins act as co-enzymes and are required for normal growth, nerve and brain function and reproduction.

### B1(thiamine)

B1(thiamine) is required by the body as a component of the enzymes that control carbohydrate **metabolism**. Thiamine is widely distributed in both animal and vegetable food. Deficiency causes beri-beri, a condition where there is muscle wasting and paralysis.

### B2 (riboflavin)

B2 (riboflavin) is required for aerobic respiration. It is found in leafy vegetables, fish and eggs. Deficiency causes dermatitis and skin lesions.

### B5 (pantotenic acid)

B5 (pantotenic acid) is required for the release of energy from fat and carbohydrate **metabolism**. It is found in animal and plant sources. Deficiency causes anaemia and vomiting.

### B12

B12 is needed for correct red blood cell formation. It is found in red meat, liver and kidney. Deficiency causes anaemia.

## Vitamin C (ascorbic acid)

Vitamin C is needed for the maintenance of healthy tissue; man is unable to form his own supply. It is widely distributed in foods, and the main sources are citrus fruits and leafy vegetables. Deficiency causes bleeding from small blood vessels into the gums, wounds heal more slowly and scurvy may develop.

# Minerals

Minerals are widely available in foods in the United Kingdom. They are required in small amounts and have many functions in the body. Calcium, iron, fluoride phosphorus, sodium, potassium, magnesium, chlorine and zinc are all required in the diet for a variety of reasons. Why do you think fluoride is required?

## Minerals

| Mineral | Function | Source | Possible result of deficiency |
|---------|----------|--------|-------------------------------|
| Calcium | Formation and maintenance of bone, blood clotting, muscle contraction | Milk, cheese, tinned fish (e.g. tuna, salmon), nuts | Acceleration of osteoporosis, poor skeletal growth, delayed blood clotting, muscle spasm |
| Chlorine | Nerve and muscle activity | Cheese, cooking salt | Rare |
| Copper | Co-enzyme for many enzymes including iron absorption | Green vegetables, fish, oysters | Rare |

*Continued overleaf*

*Minerals continued*

| Mineral | Function | Source | Possible result of deficiency |
|---|---|---|---|
| Fluoride | Helps prevent tooth decay | Drinking water, toothpaste | Tooth decay |
| Iodine | Part of thyroxine hormone secreted by the thyroid gland | Seafood, iodised table salt | Goitre |
| Iron | Formation of red blood cells, many roles in metabolism | Red meat, pulses, green vegetables | Iron deficiency, anaemia |
| Magnesium | Energy, metabolism | Most foods | Rare |
| Phosphorus | Skeletal formation | Most foods | Rare |
| Potassium | Balance of body fluids | Most foods | Rare |
| Sodium | Nerve and muscle activity | Cooking salt | Muscle cramps |
| Zinc | Tissue repair, growth and development | Most foods | Rare |

## Dietary guidelines

There are still some uncertainties about the modifications of diet which are necessary to a healthy lifestyle, but the evidence is becoming steadily more certain. The essential feature of the COMA recommendations shown opposite are as follows:

- The total fat intake should be reduced to 35 per cent of food energy, representing about 80 g a day.
- Saturated fat intake should be no more than 15 per cent of food energy.
- The ratio of polyunsaturated to saturated fats should be increased to about 0.45.
- Fibre-rich carbohydrate (bread, cereals, fruit, and vegetables) should be increased to compensate for reduced fat intake.

A twentieth-century phenomenon has been a shift to a higher fat and sugar content and lower fibre content in the diet. Sodium intake and alcohol consumption has also rapidly increased in recent years. The guidelines are therefore aimed at reducing the high fat (especially saturated fat) content and refined carbohydrate (sugar), and increasing the fibre intake. The overall aim is to prevent the 'diseases of industrialisation' or of affluence. These diseases include obesity, coronary heart disease, hypertension, diabetes mellitus, dental caries, various cancers, large bowel disorders, gallstones, haemorrhoids and varicose veins.

## Activity 4.2

Spend between five and ten minutes making a list of all the different types of food you have eaten in the past 24 hours. Now look at each of these foods and decide whether they are composed mostly of fat, carbohydrate or protein. Try to work out the approximate percentage of each of these major classes of food in your diet over the last 24 hours. Now compare your diet to that recommended by the nutritional guidelines above.

**Summary of dietary guidelines**

| Dietary component | Current estimated intake | NACNE proposals Short term | NACNE proposals Long term | COMA recommendations |
|---|---|---|---|---|
| Energy intake | | Recommended adjustment to the types of food eaten; increased exercise programme so that adult body weight is achieved and/or maintained within the optimal limits of weight-for-height | | |
| Total fat (% of total energy) | 42 | 34 | 30 | 35 |
| Saturated fat (% of total energy) | 20 | 15 | 10 | 15 |
| Polyunsaturated fat (% of total energy) | 5; P:S ratio 0:23 | No specific recommendation | | Increase P:S ratio to approx 0.45 |
| Cholesterol (mg/day) | 350–450 | No specific recommendation | | |
| Sucrose (kg/head/year) | 38 | 34 | 20 | The intake of simple sugars should not be increased |
| Fibre (g/head/day) | 20 | 25 | 30 | No specific recommendation |
| Salt intake (g/head/day) | 8–12 | 7–11 | 5–9 | Salt intake should not be increased. Ways should be sought to decrease the intake. The amount added in and after cooking should be decreased immediately |
| Alcohol (% of total energy) | 4–9 | 5 | 4 | Excessive intake should be avoided on general health grounds |
| Protein (% of total energy) | 11 | No recommendation | | No recommendation, but highlighting that animal protein tends to be associated with saturated fatty acids and vegetable protein with dietary fibre |

*Source: Nutrition Matters for Practice Nurses, ed. A Leeds, P Judd, B Lewis (John Libbey & Company Ltd)*

# The digestive system

Food is vital for life. It is the raw material that builds our body and supplies energy for our daily activities. Food as we eat it is not in a suitable state for use as an energy source. It must be broken down into **nutrient** molecules so that it can be utilised by the body. This work is carried out by the digestive system.

A healthy digestive system is essential to maintaining life. It converts the food into the raw materials that build and fuel our body's cells. The digestive system takes in food, breaks it down into nutrient molecules, absorbs these molecules into the blood stream and then excretes the indigestible remains not required by the body.

The organs of the digestive system are discussed in two main groups: the alimentary canal and the accessory organs of digestion.

## The alimentary canal

The alimentary canal, also called the gastrointestinal tract (GI), is a continuous, coiled, hollow muscular tube that winds its way through the ventral body cavity and is open to the external environment at both ends.

The organs of the alimentary canal are:
- the mouth
- the pharynx
- the oesophagus
- the stomach
- the small intestine
- the large intestine.

## The accessory organs of digestion

The accessory organs are:
- the teeth
- the tongue
- the gallbladder.

The digestive glands are:
- the salivary glands
- the liver
- the pancreas.

These glands produce saliva, bile and enzymes, which contribute to the breakdown of the food.

## Digestive processes

Food is prepared for consumption by the digestive processes:
- Ingestion, mastication and swallowing: ingestion (the taking in of food) and mastication are functions performed by the mouth and teeth, aided by the tongue. In the mouth the food is chewed and mixed with saliva. Chewing reduces the food to suitable sizes for swallowing and increases the available surface area for enzymes to act on.
- Movement of food along the alimentary canal food moves along the alimentary canal by the process of peristalsis. The walls of the alimentary canal contain circular and longitudinal muscle fibres. The circular muscles, by alternately contracting and relaxing, squeeze the food steadily forward along the alimentary canal in a wave-like movement from one organ to the next.

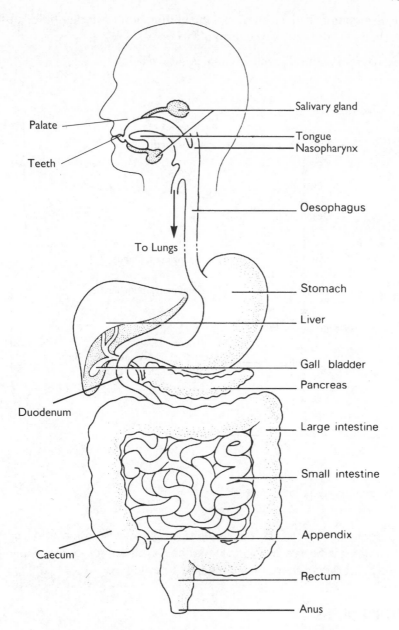

Palate

Teeth

Salivary gland

Tongue
Nasopharynx

Oesophagus

To Lungs

Stomach

Liver

Gall bladder
Pancreas

Duodenum

Large intestine

Small intestine

Appendix

Caecum

Rectum

Anus

*The digestive system and accessory organs*

- The breakdown of food by mechanical and chemical processes (digestion): mechanical digestion prepares food for chemical digestion by enzymes. Mechanical processes include chewing, mixing of food with saliva by the tongue, churning food in the stomach and mixing it with digestive juices. Chemical digestion is accomplished by enzymes secreted by various glands into the **lumen** of the alimentary canal. It is a **catabolic** process where large food molecules are broken down to their monomers (chemical building blocks), which are small enough to be absorbed into the blood stream.
- Absorption is the transport of the digested food from the alimentary canal into the cardiovascular and lymphatic systems for distribution to cells.

- Excretion and defecation are the elimination of indigestible substances from the body via the anus in the form of faeces.

A diagram of the alimentary canal is shown below.

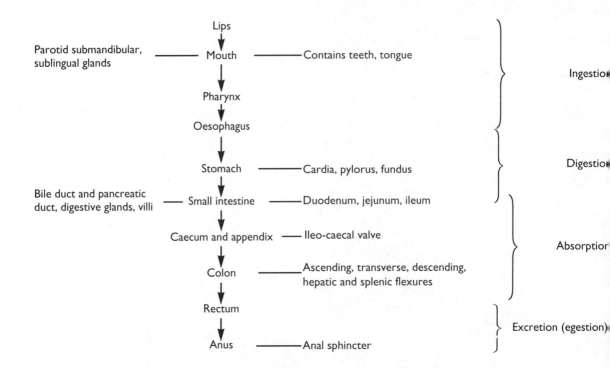

*Diagrammatic representation of the alimentary canal*

**Care point** | Abdominal pain may be the result of hunger or distension of the stomach after a heavy meal. Severe griping pain may be a symptom of food poisoning or bowel obstruction which may need medical attention.

# Specific dietary plans
## Weight-reducing diet

Overweight and obesity are the result of an excess of energy intake over expenditure. Energy requirements vary greatly among individuals, depending upon hereditary, psychological and physiological factors. Lifestyles with little physical activity and a sedentary job may also be contributory factors.

One of the most effective ways of reducing calorie intake is to reduce fat, sugars and other refined carbohydrates in the diet. By increasing complex carbohydrates, wholegrain bread, cereals, vegetables and fruit in the diet, and increasing muscular exercise, for instance walking instead of driving or taking a bus to school or work, successful weight reduction may be achieved. Eating between meals should also be avoided, especially high-energy foods such as crisps and sweets. Regular weighing and motivation to lose weight are also essential.

A number of psychological and social factors may interact to produce abnormal eating behaviour. An obese person may find themselves in a vicious circle: being depressed because of their weight, they eat for comfort, and put on more weight. Breaking the circle is difficult and an understanding of the complexities of the problems is important.

## Activity 4.3

Try to think of the factors that may motivate someone to lose weight. Make a list of these, putting them into different categories. Now try to think of factors that would keep a client motivated while on a diet. These may be different from the factors which originally motivated them to diet. Refer to a book on nutrition from the reading list to help you with this activity.

### An example of a weight-reducing diet

| | |
|---|---|
| Breakfast | Half a grapefruit |
| | Wholemeal toast with low-fat spread used sparingly |
| | Tea/coffee with semi-skimmed or skimmed milk – no added sugar |
| Mid-morning break | Apple or other fruit |
| | Low-calorie drink |
| Lunch | Chicken salad with low-calorie or no added dressing |
| | Tea/coffee as before |
| Dinner | Grilled fish |
| | Boiled potatoes |
| | Selection of vegetables |
| | Fruit or low fat yoghurt |
| | Fruit drink |

A person following a weight-reducing diet should be as inventive as they like, but remember to reduce the total calorie intake over 24 hours, and aim to lose weight at the rate of about one to two pounds per week.

Food to think carefully about before eating includes:

- sugar, glucose, sweets and honey
- cakes, scones, puddings, and pastry
- fried food which has been coated in batter or crumbs
- fried bread or fried potatoes.

## Activity 4.4

Choose any packaged food and examine the label for information about the following:

- the main ingredient
- the net quantity
- any additives, for example flavour enhancer.

Compare it with a similar product which is advertised as having reduced calories. Mayonnaise or yoghurt could be used for comparisons. What do you discover about the food labelling?

## Vegetarian diets

The underlying requirement for vegetarians, as for anyone else, is to eat a sufficien
amount of varied foods to meet energy and other nutritional needs. There are three
basic types of vegetarians:

- lacto-ovo-vegetarians: a mixed diet of both plant and animal sources is eaten. Meat
  especially red meat is excluded. Dairy products, eggs, fish and occasionally poultry are included in the diet. There are normally no nutritional problems.
- lacto-vegetarians: a basic diet of plant food supplemented by dairy produce is
  eaten. Milk and milk products such as cheese, with a varied diet of grains
  legumes, seeds, nuts, fruit and vegetables in quantities sufficient to meet energy
  needs provides a balanced intake.
- vegans: vegans use no food from animal sources, and depend entirely on plant food
  grains, fruit, legumes, nuts, seeds and vegetables. There is very little fat in this diet
  The food combinations need to be carefully planned to prevent deficiencies.

*Care point*

Care workers may need to offer dietary advice to some of the vulnerable groups
of people in society, such as elderly people living on a low income or young adolescent girls who are excessively figure-conscious. Pressure from peer groups and
the media may make both boys and girls follow an unhealthy diet.
Reasons for choosing and eating particular foods may include cultural influences,
health status, family habits, the need of the individual, age, sex, work, lifestyle,
income and availability.

## Activity 4.5

Choose one of the following individuals or groups and plan a balanced diet for them
over five days:

- a group of 8–9-year-old schoolchildren
- an adolescent girl or boy
- a woman expecting her first child
- an elderly person living alone.

Consider social, cultural and economical influences on diet as well as individual preferences. Again, you may need to refer to a textbook of nutrition to help you with
this activity. Include this work in your portfolio.

# Food production

The Common Agricultural Policy (CAP) has influenced the production of food in
Europe for many years. Some aspects of this policy have favoured healthy eating but
most people are more familiar with the surpluses that have accumulated, and the
work undertaken to reduce them. There is no common European legislation; each
country has its own guidelines. Some work undertaken on nutrition labelling is an
attempt to standardise and harmonise policies throughout Europe.

## Availabilty

Most of the food we eat, from plants or animals, is cultivated on farms. The development of a nation-wide transport network in the nineteenth century made it possible

to transport food around the country. Perishable goods such as soft fruit and milk could be on sale in London four or five hours after being delivered to a station in Cornwall.

# Food sources

The human diet can include the following:
- meat, normally regarded as the edible parts (muscle and offal) of the animal. The animals eaten are those which consume mainly grass and other arable crops, for example, cattle, sheep and pigs.
- poultry, which has become a major meat-producing species.
- fish and other seafoods; these have been an important part of human diet since earliest times.
- non-meat products (see below).

All the above animals, including fish, are converters, that is they utilise green vegetable material with varying efficiency to produce protein.

## Meat

In the United Kingdom the annual consumption of meat and meat products, which represent about one-tenth of the total household expenditure on food, amounts to approximately £1000 million per year at retail prices. Consumer demand is now for leaner meat (venison is becoming increasingly popular) in waste-free cuts which are easy and quick to prepare.

The future of meat and meat products will depend mainly on consumer demand and the prices at which they can be profitably produced. As living standards rise so also does the consumption of meat.

## Poultry

Poultry farming is widespread throughout the world. China, USA, the former Soviet Union, France, UK and many others produce millions of birds per year. There are many large commercial organisations in which thousands of birds are kept under the most modern systems of management. Much effort has been put into the breeding of poultry for both egg and meat production. Poultry meat production in the UK is mainly broilers, supplemented by cockerels, capons, and hens together with turkeys, ducks, geese, guinea fowl, and some game species such as grouse, partridges, pheasants and quail. Ostrich farming has recently been introduced into England.

## Fish

There is along tradition of seafaring in the British Isles. Ports such as Fleetwood, Grimsby and Great Yarmouth see fishing vessels leave regularly to fish the rich waters around the UK. Fleets of factory ships freeze the fish or process it into animal feed as soon as it is caught. This increasing efficiency over the last 20 years has, however, resulted in overfishing; herring has been fished almost to extinction in the North Atlantic and cod and haddock are becoming increasingly rare. (Pollution of the sea is also responsible for depletion of stocks in some areas.)

Aquaculture, fish farming is becoming more widespread with salmon and trout reared under controlled conditions to supplement the natural supply; about 10 per cent of the world's fish are now produced in this way. The United Nations would like this figure increased to 15 or 20 per cent by the year 2000.

## Non-meat products

Demand from vegetarians has led to health foods without meat content coming on to the market. There have been attempts to increase the use of potentially cheaper, non-meat proteins in human foods, for example vegetable protein derived mainly from soya beans, cotton seed, ground nuts, sunflower, rape and sesame.

Three main classes of vegetable protein products, usually based on soya, are meat analogue, textured vegetable protein and extended meat. These all vary in composition and production costs.

Meat analogue is soya protein spun into filaments and bound with more protein such as egg albumin. Textured vegetable protein may be meal concentrates or protein isolator combined with carbohydrates in the form of starch. Extended meat is a mixture of vegetable and meat protein which is subjected to normal heat processing; various flavours, colours and even fat can be added.

## Production methods

Farming is one of the most important industries in the United Kingdom and Europe, producing most of the food the population needs. For thousands of years farmers have raised animals for meat, milk and eggs, all important sources of protein. Farms may be:

- mixed, producing crops and animals
- producing cattle for meat
- dairy, producing cattle for milk
- arable, producing cereals, such as wheat, barley, maize, millet or sorghum.

Intensive in farming followed specialisation; expensive machinery and chemicals are used to produce very high yields, even surpluses which have to be stored.

Technology is used in the production of livestock: pigs and chickens are housed in units where the temperature, ventilation, food and water supplies are monitored and controlled by computer systems. Chicken and pork have been produced more efficiently and cheaply by these methods.

Concern about the welfare of the animals and the cruelty of these methods has, however, been expressed by many people and organisations, along with concern at the use of chemicals used to protect crops: insecticides, herbicides and fungicides. Many farms are returning to traditional organic methods, producing crops and livestock without the use of chemicals. Natural methods avoid costly fertilisers but are labour intensive and the smaller quantities produced result in more expensive products.

## Future influences

Factors such as the consumption of meat, feed-conversion efficiency, land use and availability, consumer taste, price to consumers, diet, attitudes of people to meat production methods, use of protein from non-animal sources will all play a part in determining future demands.

## Food hygiene

Hygiene is the science of preserving health. We can never afford to relax standards of food hygiene. The aim of food hygiene is the production of food that is both safe and

clean. The important features to remember are:
- animal products must be initially safe before they enter the food industry or other establishments such as hospitals, schools, hotels, restaurants, nursing homes and home kitchens
- the hygiene of those working in the food industry must be unquestionable
- the conditions of storage must be appropriate to the type of food.

Hygiene is much more than cleanliness; it includes all practices, precautions and procedures involved in:
- protecting food from risk of contamination of any kind
- preventing any organisms multiplying to an extent which would expose consumers to risk or result in premature decomposition of food.

The cost of poor hygiene is extremely high with the incidence of food poisoning rising every year.

## Establishing and maintaining food hygiene

Good hygiene practice is essential in food factories. The buildings are specially designed and built for particular purposes with interior smooth surfaces that are non-porous, easily cleaned and not vulnerable to chemical attack by detergents or disinfectants. The lighting, temperature and humidity are all carefully controlled. A good water supply and a careful cleaning schedule management are required.

### Preparation
It is important to prevent the contamination of foods. During preparation the utensils and equipment used should be kept clean by regular washing and rinsing. Dishwashing machines are usually available in cafes, schools, community homes and hospitals.

The cooking process destroys bacteria present in raw food. Raw foods should be kept apart from cooked foods to prevent any risk of contamination by bacteria. Any food known to be contaminated must be disposed off safely.

It is important to remember that food should be kept scrupulously clean and free from any noxious materials that may be in the atmosphere, such as insecticide sprays, for example.

> **Presentation of food**
>
> The presentation of food is very important. Nicely presented food is more appetising and pleasing to the client. Small portions of well-prepared food are appreciated, particularly by the elderly. Clients will also appreciate having a choice.

*Care point*

## Food poisoning

Eating contaminated food can lead to food poisoning, an infection of the gastro-intestinal tract which may present as diarrhoea and vomiting. The organisms that are commonly responsible for this type of infection are salmonella, escherichia coli and shigella. Food poisoning is a notifiable disease and, as stated above, one which appears to be increasing.

**Care point** ▶
As a carer you must be very careful not to serve food that may harm your client in any way. What would you do if you opened a carton of milk that had an unpleasant smell, but the expiry date was still several days away?

## Personal hygiene

All people who prepare and handle food have a moral obligation to observe basic principles of **personal hygiene**. Take care of your general health by having regular check-ups. It is important when preparing food to take special care to wash the hands thoroughly before handling any food.

## Healthy eating

Individual attitudes and knowledge about nutrition are complex. People with higher levels of education and younger people are usually more aware of the importance of nutrition in maintaining general health. There are some areas of confusion about healthy eating which can only be resolved with better education and a better understanding of the food we eat.

The main reasons for making changes to a healthy diet are to keep healthy, help control weight, and prevent diseases later on in life. Experimenting with food can also be fun!

## Twenty questions

1   What is the major dietary threat to health?

2   Describe the cultural influences on food choice.

3   How would you recognise signs of poor nutrition?

4   Define a healthy diet.

5   What sort of milk do you usually have?

6   What type of bread do you usually have?

7   What happens to proteins in the body?

8   Name the types of information on a food label.

9   Describe the process of peristalsis.

10   Which organs are accessory organs of digestion?

11   Is chocolate good for you? Give reasons for your answer.

12   How often do you eat fresh green vegetables?

13   What is the function of fibre in the diet?

14   How would you advise a friend who wishes to lose weight?

15   What are the diseases of affluence?

16   How could we help prevent them?

17   Can diet alone prevent these diseases occurring?

18 How are eggs produced in the UK?

19 Which methods are used for producing chicken?

20 Why is it important to wash your hands before handling food?

## Quick concepts

| | |
|---|---|
| **Anabolism** | Building up of new cells from simple molecules, a process requiring energy |
| **Carbohydrate** | An organic compound containing carbon, hydrogen and oxygen |
| **Catabolism** | Breaking down of complex molecules in food into simpler molecules to produce energy |
| **Communal hygiene** | Measures taken to supply the community with pure food and water |
| **Disaccharide** | A sugar which yields two molecules of monosaccharide on hydrolysis |
| **Lumen** | The space or cavity within an artery, vein, intestine or tube |
| **Metabolism** | The constant use by the body of nutrients as a result of tissue activity |
| **Monosaccharide** | A simple sugar |
| **Nutrient** | Biochemical substance used by the body which must be supplied in adequate amounts in food |
| **Nutrition** | The process by which food is assimilated into the body for nourishment |
| **Nutritional status** | The state of health produced by the balance between requirement and intake of nutrients |
| **Personal hygiene** | Measures taken by the individual to preserve their own health |
| **Polysaccharide** | A carbohydrate containing a large number of monosaccharide groups |

## Supplementary reading

Bell, S and Carter, A, *Food in Focus*, John Wiley & Sons Ltd, Chichester, 1988

COMA, *Diet and Cardiovascular Disease*, HMSO, 1984

COMA, *Dietary Reference Values for Food Energy and Nutrients in the United Kingdom*, HMSO, 1991

The Committee of Medical Aspects of Food Policy, Report on the above title, HMSO, 1991

Gregory, J, Foster, K, Taylor, H, and Wiseman, M, *The Dietary and Nutritional Survey of British Adults*, HMSO, 1990

Johnson, A, *Factory Farming*, Blackwell, 1991

Report on Health and Social Subjects, Department of Health

Rudge, C, *The Food Connection, The BBC Guide to Healthy Eating*, BBC, 1985

Stockley, L, *The Promotion of Healthier Eating: a Basis for Action*, Health Education Authority, 1993

Tortora, GJ, Anagnostakos, NP, *Principles of Anatomy and Physiology*, Harper and Row, New York, 1987

A discussion paper on *Proposals For Nutrition Guidelines for Health Education in Britain*, National Advisory Committee on Nutrition Education, Health Education Authority, 1983

# 5 Maintaining physical health and well-being through exercise

## What is covered in this chapter

- The muscular system and the effects of exercise
- The cardio-vascular system and the effects of exercise
- The respiratory system and the effects of exercise
- Exercise, physical health and mental well-being
- Exercise for different client groups

## Introduction

In June 1992, the Health Education Authority and the Sports Council published the results of the most comprehensive survey to measure fitness levels and physical activity patterns ever undertaken in any country. The survey showed that although the vast majority of the population of England believe themselves to be fit, one third of men and two thirds of women are unable to continue walking at a reasonable pace up a slight slope without becoming breathless. This is because seven out of ten men and eight out of ten women do not take sufficient regular exercise to achieve health benefit.

The benefits of exercise and the detrimental effects of insufficient exercise are evident. People who have taken up regular exercise have shown increased levels of fitness. The effects of exercise on the body (and mind) are discussed in this chapter. The following points are generally accepted.

- Reduced physical activity in children is linked with risk factors such as high blood pressure, high fat levels in the blood and obesity.

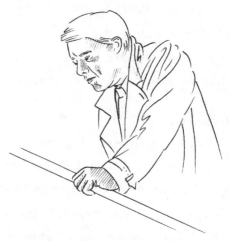

*One third of men are unable to continue walking at a reasonable pace up a slight slope without becoming breathless*

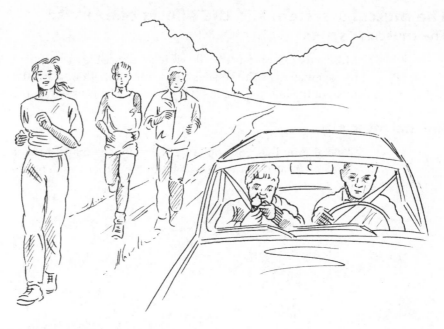

*Exercise is beneficial to everyone*

- Exercise is known to play a significant part in lessening the risk of coronary heart disease.
- Exercise can help to prevent the loss of bone mass associated with osteoporosis. It may also reduce the stiffness of connective tissues associated with advancing age.
- Older people have demonstrated an increased ability to concentrate, even a short time after starting a regular exercise programme.
- There is some evidence to suggest that exercise enhances the ability of the body to produce certain nutrients.

## Activity 5.1

Make a list of all the sports and leisure centres, gyms, swimming pools, squash clubs, tennis clubs and any other facilities in your area that offer exercise-related activities.

Pay a visit, preferably to a centre that offers a wide range of activities, and evaluate its effectiveness in encouraging and motivating people to exercise. List the ways in which this is achieved, for example, are the staff friendly and welcoming? You may find that this activity encourages you to start exercising, if you do not do so already!

You could carry out a more detailed study, but will need to seek permission of the centre manager first. You might organise your study as follows:
- Prepare a questionnaire for existing users of the facility to evaluate the quality of the service offered.
- Observe the number of people arriving and leaving for information regarding patterns of use.
- Investigate whether any particular sections of the community are catered for, for example, older people, or people who have a disability. Is there any special equipment available that could benefit such groups of people? Are there wheelchair ramps?
- Is fitness for children and young people promoted?

# The muscular system and the effects of exercise
## The muscular system

Muscle tissue consists of cells which are capable of contraction. Skeletal muscle works in conjunction with the skeleton, while smooth and cardiac muscle produces movement of the internal organs. This chapter is concerned mainly with skeletal muscle.

## Skeletal muscle

Skeletal muscle is controlled by the voluntary part of the nervous system. It is composed of striated (striped) cells bound together by connective tissue. These cells form muscle fibres.

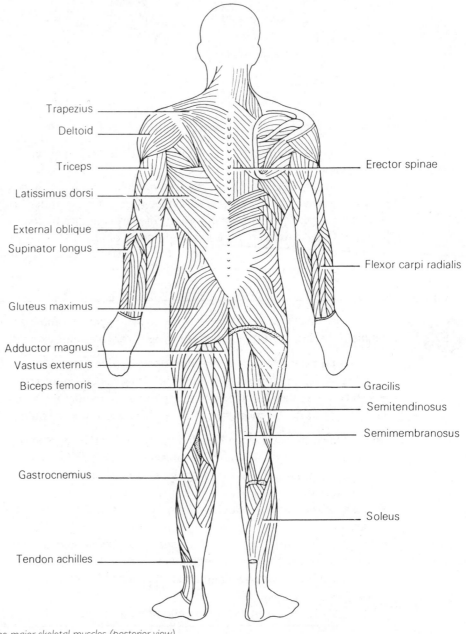

Trapezius

Deltoid

Triceps

Latissimus dorsi

External oblique

Supinator longus

Gluteus maximus

Adductor magnus

Vastus externus

Biceps femoris

Gastrocnemius

Tendon achilles

Erector spinae

Flexor carpi radialis

Gracilis

Semitendinosus

Semimembranosus

Soleus

*The major skeletal muscles (posterior view)*

## Activity 5.2

Examine a small piece of lean meat: if you tease it apart, it will reveal the existence of bundles of threadlike structures. These are muscle fibres.

### Muscle fibres

Bundles of muscle fibres are called fasciculi. An individual muscle consists of many fasciculi enveloped in a sheet of areolar tissue, which is continuous with the tendon. The tendon attaches the muscle to the bone.

Each muscle fibre is served by at least one nerve fibre. In normal use a few muscle fibres are stimulated in turn, which maintains muscle tone, even when the muscle as

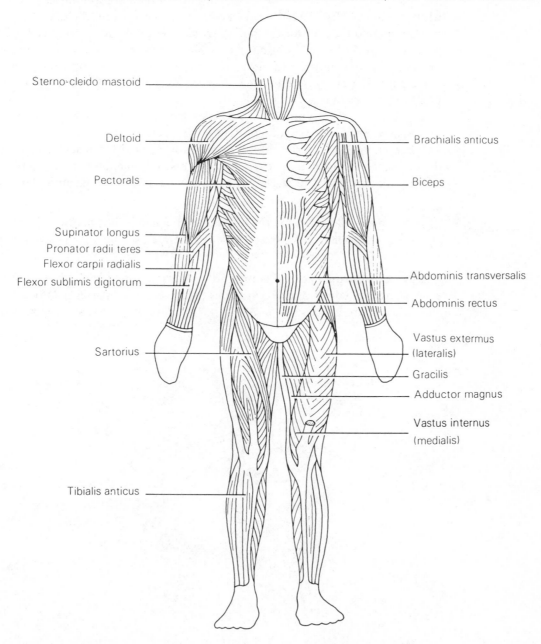

*The major skeletal muscles (anterior view)*

a whole is at rest. When many fibres are stimulated in turn (as in exercise, for example), shortening of the whole muscle results in an isotonic contraction (see page 80.)

### The blood supply to the muscles

The muscle requires an adequate blood supply for glucose and oxygen to be received. Chemical changes involving these substances release the energy that is necessary for the muscle to contract.

## Muscles during exercise

### Energy sources

The immediate source of energy in the muscle is a compound called **adenosine triphosphate** (ATP). The harder the body works, the greater the rate at which it uses energy; therefore the faster the rate at which energy must be produced. ATP can be produced quickly from creatine phosphate (a substance that is also present in the muscle), but this supply is limited and lasts for only 30 to 60 seconds before being depleted. It can be considered as a 'start-up' system, which is **anaerobic,** that is the presence of oxygen is not required.

The subsequent resynthesis of ATP depends on the breakdown of carbohydrate during **aerobic** metabolism (the presence of oxygen is required).

When energy is required rapidly, a substance called lactic acid is created. Again, this is formed under anaerobic conditions. This system allows energy to be produced very rapidly to match the high energy requirements of intensive muscular effort.

*Care point*  The build-up of lactic acid in the muscle can be painful. It is preferable to warm up gradually before strenuous exercise, and to stretch the muscles gently as well.

Energy used during exercise is primarily derived from carbohydrate. Eat plenty of complex carbohydrate about two hours before exercise: pasta, potatoes, bread, rice and bananas are good sources. Avoid simple carbohydrates, such as sweets, choco-

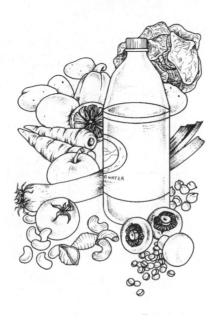

*A healthy balanced diet will help the body to function more efficiently during exercise*

late, biscuits and cakes. These will give you a short-lived energy boost, whereas complex carbohydrate will give you slow-release energy over a longer period of time.

## Summary: energy for muscular work

Adenosine triphosphate (ATP) is the immediate source of energy in the muscle. ATP is broken down to ADP (adenosine diphosphate) when energy is required. For the continuing production of energy, a cyclical process involving the resynthesis of ATP is necessary. An initial, rapid but short burst of energy can be generated by creatine phosphate, which is stored in the muscle. Glycogen is broken down to form pyruvate, which is oxidised to generate ATP. High energy requirements of intensive muscular efforts can be met by pyruvate being converted to lactic acid.

The oxidation (aerobic metabolism) process occurs within the mitochondria, specialised structures in the cells. They account for most of the oxygen consumed by the body.

If exercise is taken at a lower, prolonged intensity, it will be the aerobic system that will make the main contribution towards the creation of energy. The aerobic system is able to make use of the full range of stored energy without the inhibiting effects of lactic acid.

**Care point** ▶ Exercise should be fun, and not a chore. Clients should not have to experience 'pain for gain'. To improve levels of fitness and to help weight loss, most benefit will be gained from a sustained activity that raises the heart-rate without discomfort. This is because the aerobic system of energy production, which functions when exercise is prolonged but at a lower intensity, relies on the uptake of oxygen and the breakdown of carbohydrate, and fat from the adipose tissue of the body.

## Muscle fibre types

Some muscle fibre types are better equipped to work aerobically, and some to work anaerobically. There are three different types of muscle fibre in human skeletal muscle:
- type I: red, slow twitch or slow-oxidative
- type IIA: white, fast twitch or fast-oxidative glycolytic
- type IIB white, fast twitch or fast-glycolytic

Slow twitch fibres contract and relax slowly but they are resistant to fatigue. They have energy sources and pathways needed for endurance work.

Fast twitch fibres contract twice as fast as the slow and produce more force, but they tire quickly. Most individuals average about 50 per cent of each type. However, many marathon runners have about 80 per cent slow twitch muscle fibre type in their leg muscles, while sprinters have a high proportion of fast twitch fibre type.

It is believed that the main difference in the muscle fibres lies in the level of myoglobin. This is a protein material in the muscle that has a strong affinity for oxygen and gives the red colour. The red fibres therefore have a higher level of myoglobin than the white fibres. The higher myoglobin level in the red fibres allows them to have a high metabolic capacity for aerobic metabolism.

## Types of muscular contraction

The development of muscular strength involves a muscle, or group of muscles, exerting a force while contracting against a resistance. This contraction involves an increase in muscle tension. There are several types of muscular contraction, which are outlined below.

### Isotonic contraction

The muscle develops tension to overcome a resistance with associated movement of body parts. Isotonic contraction is the most familiar type of contraction, used in all lifting activities.

### Isometric contraction

The isometric contraction does not result in movement about the joint axis but the muscle does develop tension. It can be observed when an attempt is made to lift an immovable object. The isometric contraction is also known as a static contraction.

### Concentric contraction

The muscle shortens and thickens. The two end attachments of the muscle, the point of origin and the point of insertion, move closer together and the angle at the joint decreases.

### Eccentric contraction

The opposite of concentric contraction. The muscle returns to its original resting length as it develops tension against resistance, for example when lowering a weight. The points of origin and insertion are drawn further apart under control.

## Activity 5.3

Imagine that you are gripping onto a 'chin-up' bar by your hands (or try it, if you visit a gym). You are just hanging, with your feet off the ground; neither pulling yourself up, nor lowering yourself down. Which type of contraction is occurring in the arm muscles which you are using to hold yourself in that position?

## Muscles after exercise

Strength training acts as a stimulus by placing stress on a muscle, or group of muscles. As a result of this metabolic and physiological stress certain adaptations take place within the muscle. These adaptations are in the form of growth modifications made to meet the exercise demands placed on the muscle tissue. They take place during the rest and recovery phase, when protein synthesis increases to build the structural components of the muscle. Protein synthesis takes from 24 to 48 hours.

**Care point**

Anyone starting weight training should train on alternate days, or work on alternate muscle groups on different days, or alternate cardio-vascular activity (running, cycling, rowing, stepping, etc.) with weight training. Lifting weights with 'cold' muscles should be avoided; warming up first by doing some form of cardio-vascular exercise is essential. The guidance of a qualified fitness teacher should always be sought before beginning any exercise programme.

## The benefits of strength training

The benefits of strength training can be summarised as follows:
• individual muscle fibres increase in diameter following strength training; this is caused by an increase in the number of myofibrils per fibre

- a possible improvement in the nerve pathways and the transmission of impulses to the muscles
- an increased supply of blood capillaries within the muscle; this occurs so that adequate oxygen and nutrients can be supplied to the enlarged muscle fibres
- growth and toughening of the connective tissue that surrounds each muscle fibre, the bundles of fibres and the muscle itself; this includes tendons and ligaments
- reduction in the amount of fat within the muscles.

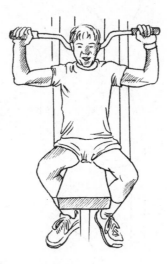

*Strength training has several benefits*

# The cardio-vascular system and the effects of exercise

## The heart and circulation

The heart is completely divided in order to keep oxygenated and deoxygenated blood separate. As a general rule, arteries transport oxygenated blood, and veins carry deoxygenated blood, the only exceptions being the pulmonary arteries and veins.

Arteries have strong, muscular walls, whereas veins have comparatively little elasticity or muscle. The pressure of blood in the arteries is therefore higher than in the veins. The force exerted against the walls of the arteries is referred to as blood pressure.

Arterioles are the smallest arteries which break up into a number of minute vessels called capillaries. These consist of a single-cell layer through which small-molecule substances can pass.

Blood in the arteries flows in spurts which are synchronous with the heart beat. The wave of contraction which passes along an artery wall is called a pulse, which can be felt in many places where the vessels are sufficiently superficial.

## Activity 5.4

Pulse rate is usually counted in the radial artery. Using three fingers (not your thumb) of one hand, find your radial pulse, which you should be able to locate on your arm near the base of the thumb of the other hand. Try counting your pulse by timing it for one minute.

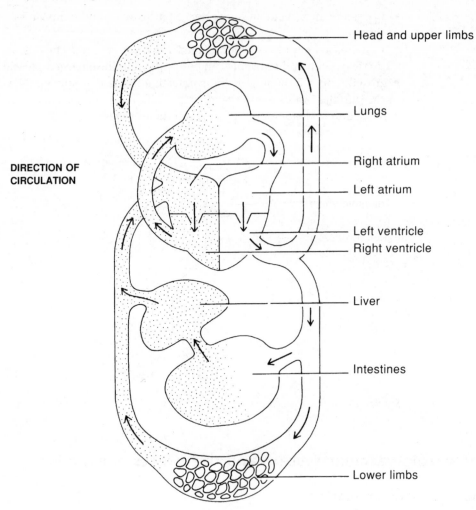

Head and upper limbs

Lungs

Right atrium

Left atrium

Left ventricle

Right ventricle

Liver

Intestines

Lower limbs

**DIRECTION OF
CIRCULATION**

*The circulation*

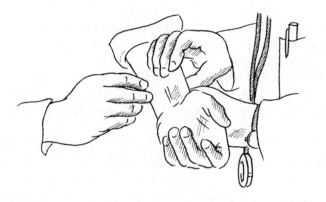

*Taking the radial pulse*

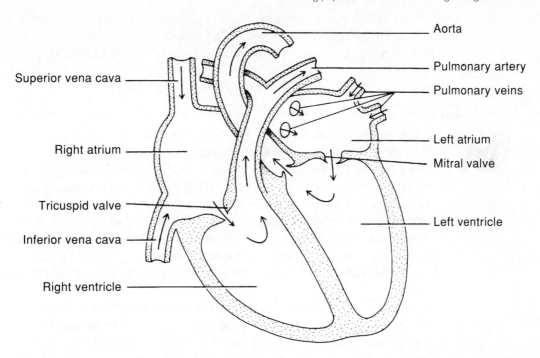

Aorta

Pulmonary artery

Pulmonary veins

Superior vena cava

Left atrium

Mitral valve

Right atrium

Tricuspid valve

Left ventricle

Inferior vena cava

Right ventricle

*The four cavities of the heart*

The heart is divided into four chambers: two ventricles and two atria. Blood vessels are connected to each chamber. The direction of the flow of blood is maintained by valves.

## The cardio-vascular system during exercise

During exercise, the skeletal muscles require more oxygen and glucose, which is transported to them via the blood. Cardiac output (and, therefore, the pulse rate) and blood pressure rise and there is redeployment in the capillary circulation (from other parts of the body) to ensure adequate supplies.

Because blood transports oxygen, the changes that occur are interrelated with the functions of the respiratory system.

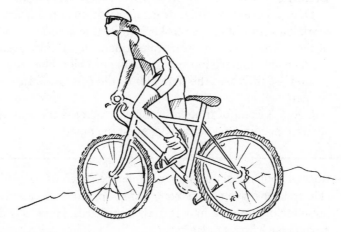

*Cycling is one form of aerobic exercise*

Under the heading *Muscles During Exercise* (page 78) it was explained that prolonged, low-intensity exercise uses the aerobic system of energy production. Increased exercise intensity results in an accumulation of lactic acid in the blood. Lactic acid is both an energy carrier and a metabolic by-product of intense effort. Aerobic exercise is defined as exercise below the point where blood lactic acid levels begin to rise.

## Activity 5.5

If you do not already follow an exercise programme, you may need to consult your GP before carrying out this experiment.

Use a running machine or the local park for this activity. Warm up first by walking, gently mobilising your joints and stretching. Proceed from a slow to a brisk walk. Break into a light jog, and gradually increase your speed until the effort becomes uncomfortable, your breathing is deep and rapid, and you begin to doubt your ability to continue. Everything up to this point has been aerobic, or in the presence of oxygen. If you continued to increase exercise intensity beyond this point, you would change to anaerobic or non-oxidative exercise, which is not recommended for this activity!

Remember to reduce the intensity of the exercise as gradually as you increased it; do not stop suddenly, however tempting this may be. The body needs to adapt to its resting state gradually. Reverse, therefore, the preceding process by gradually reducing your speed until you return to a slow walk.

**Care point** ▷ Aerobic exercise should be relatively pleasant and relaxing, not unpleasant and painful. It should be possible to carry on a conversation during moderate aerobic exercise.

## The cardio-vascular system after exercise

Aerobic fitness is the ability to take in, transport and utilise oxygen. Regular aerobic exercise will improve aerobic fitness. This is because exercise overloads oxygen transport and utilisation systems, and the body adapts to the increased requirements.

### Benefits of exercise to the cardio-vascular system

Over a period of time, exercise can reduce the heart rate at rest, and at a given work load, and improve stroke volume (the amount of blood pumped with each beat of the heart). A slower heart rate equates to an improved stroke volume because the heart chambers have more time to fill with blood between beats.

Exercise increases the diameter of the coronary arteries that supply the heart with oxygen.

Over a period of time, exercise can increase the amount of haemoglobin (the substance that combines with oxygen) in the blood.

## Activity 5.6

Record your radial pulse for one minute. Then using either an aerobic step, a suitable stair or a gymnastics bench, step up and down for three minutes. Record your pulse for one minute immediately afterwards. How long does it take for you to regain your resting pulse rate?

## Activity 5.7

Calculate your target training zone: the level of increase in your pulse rate during exercise, which depends on how fit you are. To calculate it, subtract your age from 220. Your target training zone is between 60 and 90 per cent of the result. However, if you are not very fit, you should restrict the raising of your pulse rate to between 60 and 80 per cent of the figure reached.

# The respiratory system and the effects of exercise

## The respiratory system

Respiration is the process whereby oxygen is obtained and used for the oxidation of food materials to liberate energy and to produce carbon dioxide and water as waste materials.

### Internal respiration

Internal respiration is the chain of chemical processes which take place in every living cell to free energy for its vital activities.

### External respiration

External respiration is the means by which oxygen is obtained from the environment and carbon dioxide is released into it. This process is referred to as gaseous exchange and takes place in the lungs. The bloodstream carries oxygen away from, and carbon dioxide to, the lungs. Air reaches the lungs through the respiratory passages. The system dealing with external respiration involves nasal passages, pharynx, larynx, trachea, bronchi and lungs (see the illustration below) in addition to the muscles involved in making the breathing movements.

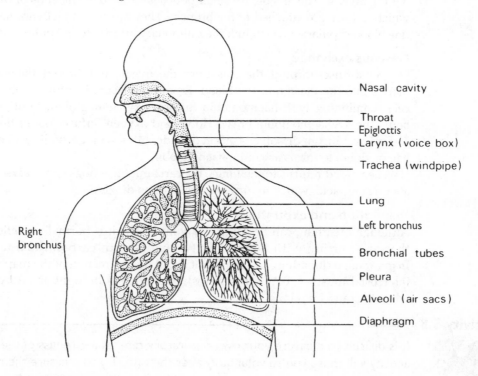

*The respiratory system*

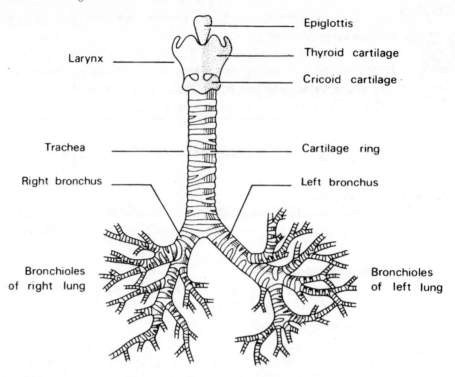

*The respiratory passages*

### The alveoli

Oxygen from the air in the lungs dissolves in the thin film of moisture on the cells lining the **alveoli**. The alveoli are small pouches situated at the ends of the bronchioles, which in turn, are attached to the bronchi. They are close to a dense network of very fine blood capillaries which link the pulmonary arteries to the pulmonary veins.

### Gaseous exchange

Oxygen diffuses through the cells lining the alveoli, and through the walls of the capillaries into the plasma of the blood. From the plasma it diffuses into the red blood cells, combining with haemoglobin to form oxyhaemoglobin. In other parts of the body, the oxyhaemoglobin breaks down and oxygen diffuses out of the blood, while carbonic acid from dissolved carbon dioxide diffuses in. Carbonic acid combines with haemoglobin to form carbaminohaemoglobin.

When blood returns to the lungs, the carbaminohaemoglobin breaks down to liberate carbonic acid, which in turn liberates carbon dioxide.

### Inspiration and expiration

Although breathing can be controlled voluntarily, it is normally a reflex action with the rate varying with body activity, that is with carbon dioxide production. Inspiration, or breathing in, is brought about by contraction of the diaphragm and the intercostal muscles (between the ribs); expiration is brought about by elastic recoil when the muscles relax.

## Activity 5.8

It is difficult to measure your own respiratory rate, as awareness of the intended activity will cause you to voluntarily alter the rate. Try to measure the respiratory rate of a another person, at rest, preferably when they are unaware! Count the rise and fall of the chest as one. Expect the rate to be between 16–22 per minute for a healthy adult.

## The respiratory system during exercise

During exercise, increased demands are made upon the respiratory system for more circulating oxygen in the blood, so that the body can use the aerobic system of energy production. The respiratory rate will become more rapid to increase the uptake of oxygen. The degree of rapidity depends upon the aerobic fitness level of the individual. This is explained in the next section.

## The respiratory system after exercise

Exercise improves the condition and efficiency of breathing muscles so that the body can make use of more lung capacity during exercise. Aerobic exercise improves total lung capacity in at least two ways:
- by increasing the inspiratory reserve (the amount of air that can be breathed in with maximum effort)
- by reducing the residual volume (the amount of air left in the lungs after breathing out with maximum effort)
- by increasing the vital capacity (which is the tidal volume – the amount of air breathed in and out when a person breathes normally – plus the inspiratory and expiratory reserve volumes – the air breathed in and out with more effort).

Residual volume increases with age and inactivity. The decline in total lung capacity eventually reduces the capacity for exercise. However, aerobic exercise can halt or even reverse the decline and ensure adequate respiration throughout life Exercise increases the maximum amount of air that can be breathed per minute. It also enhances the efficiency of the process, so fewer breaths are needed to move the same volume of air. Slower, deeper breaths are more efficient because they allow better penetration of air into the alveolar sacs and more time for oxygen to enter the circulation. Exercise improves diffusion of oxygen from the lung into the capillaries of the pulmonary system. Exercise can help to reduce body fat percentage, and so improve body shape, especially when attention is also paid to dietary intake.

# Exercise, physical health and mental well-being

## Stress management

Exercise may help to reduce stress by enabling the individual to channel stress-related energy. In addition, the physical health gains from exercise may help an individual (who is healthier and more energetic) to manage stress more effectively.

## Other benefits

The Sports Council promotes exercise as having the following benefits:
- helping people to feel good in mind and body
- providing fun and improving social life, by meeting people pursuing similar goals
- promoting suppleness and mobility
- strengthening muscles, joints and bones

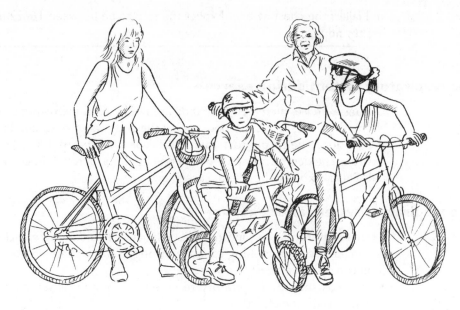

*Cycling can benefit all age groups*

- improving blood circulation
- improving the functioning of just about all the systems of the body.

### Co-ordination

Exercise such as aerobics can improve motor co-rdination with the blend of physical movement and simple choreography. Different client groups could benefit from aerobics presented in a form appropriate to their needs and abilities.

**Activity 5.9**

Collect some evidence of the benefits of exercise by keeping an exercise journal. You can only do this if you embark upon a programme of regular, planned exercise! If you decide to start exercising by joining a health club or sports centre, for example, make sure that you obtain guidance from an appropriately qualified instructor. There are recognised RSA and Sports Council approved qualifications relating to weight training, circuit training and exercise to music.

First, you need to record some base-line measurements. Use the following as a guide:

- weight
- body measurements (upper arms, waist, hips, upper legs, chest).

Try a step test (see section on the cardio-vascular system). Record your resting pulse-rate, then the pulse rate following the three-minute test, then the length of time that it takes to return to your resting pulse rate.

You may use some of the machinery as measurement tools, if you begin to use a gym; for example, a running machine should tell you how many kilometres you have covered, in how many minutes.

You may find somebody who can measure your body fat percentage (this is likely to be a qualified fitness instructor), using callipers.

Do not revisit these measurements too frequently, as you may lose motivation if you do not see results. If you take planned exercise at least three times per week, try recording any physical changes once a month. Increase the time to six or eight weeks if you are not seeing any significant changes. Some of the changes will, of course, depend upon your personal goals. For some, these will include weight loss; for others the priority may be increased fitness, or increased muscle tone, or size. A good fitness instructor will take into account your personal goals when planning an exercise programme.

When completing your exercise journal, make note of how you feel after exercise (not immediately after, but when you have showered and are relaxing), and any effects that it may have had upon your life in general; for example, do you feel less tired? More confident? More energetic?

It is worth noting that if you do not feel that you are gaining any benefit from exercise, you may need to consider other aspects of your life, for example your diet and factors that may be affecting your emotional well-being, perhaps relating to work or relationships. Optimum health requires a holistic approach.

## Exercise for different client groups

As we have seen, exercise will have a beneficial effect on the following areas:
- muscular strength
- muscular endurance
- cardiovascular fitness
- flexibility
- co-ordination.

These headings are also the factors that need to be taken into consideration when planning an exercise programme (see the section *A multi-professional approach*, page 91). Whatever the client group, it is highly likely that they can benefit from exercise.

**Care point** ▶ Medical guidance should be sought before embarking upon an exercise programme with a client, as their individual health needs may limit the type of activity that they can safely pursue.

## Exercise for the elderly

Some of the benefits of exercise to the older person were mentioned in the introduction (page 75). Other benefits of exercise for this group may include the following:
- more efficient circulation, which helps to promote healing and to prevent the development of pressure sores.
- increased uptake of oxygen; improvement of respiratory functioning.
- enhanced psychological well-being (some older people are prone to becoming depressed)
- increased socialisation (some older people become isolated, either because of immobility or because of lack of social contact)

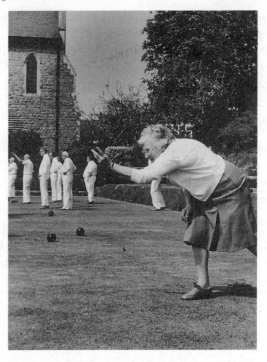

*Older people can benefit from taking exercise*

- improved function of body systems, such as the gastro-intestinal system, so that conditions such as constipation may be alleviated.
- reduction of body fat (some older people become overweight, which may affect their mobility)
- enhanced general mobility
- improved joint mobility, helping to reduce stiffness and pain
- improved muscle tone and strength, which in turn should help to prolong independence.

Obviously, there will be some constraints that will need to be taken into consideration when planning exercise for the older person.

## Exercise and disabled people

For certain client groups, the benefits of exercise may be more specific. Disability of any kind should not prevent the individual from being able to participate in some form of sport or exercise. In a study of wheelchair-bound persons using a power-ramp, climber and chin-ups to improve their fitness, men with paraplegia seemed to outperform able-bodied men in all events. Carriage-driving for disabled people can be a liberating experience and an activity at which they can compete equally with able-bodied people. The benefits of horseriding for people with a disability have been widely reported.

Sport can act as a supportive therapy for people with mental health problems and can be an important part of this client group's healthcare. Remedial gymnastics can help the rehabilitation of people with mental as well as physical health problems.

The number of sports in which disabled people take part has increased over the past twenty years. There are multiple benefits of sports for the disabled and individuals with amputations find rehabilitation in competitive sports.

# A multi-professional approach

As well as seeking medical guidance, care workers helping a client begin an exercise programme should consult as many appropriate professionals as possible.

Physiotherapists are valuable sources of information on passive and active exercise which is appropriate to individuals; they also have underlying knowledge of anatomy and physiology to support their practice.

Some fitness instructors have received additional training in working with particular client groups. It may be worth enquiring at your local sports centre to see if any of these areas of expertise are available. In addition, some sports centres have activities and equipment intended to help certain groups (for example, those with disabilities or older people) to exercise.

Factors which may affect the client and their ability to exercise must be taken onto consideration. For example, an older person might be affected by one or more of the following conditions.

## Obesity

If the client is obese, exercise will need to be of low intensity (that does not raise the heart rate too much; this will apply to many older people, not only the obese) and preferably combined with a reduced fat diet.

## Diabetes

Exercise lowers the blood sugar level. In the management of diabetes, this needs to be taken into consideration. Insulin dosage (if taken) may need to be altered, for example. A doctor should be consulted.

## Arthritis

It may be beneficial to the client with arthritis to put their joints through a range of movements. This may be helped by a warm bath.

## High blood pressure

Blood pressure (see Chapter 7) will need to be monitored if exercise is taken.

## Stroke

For a client who has had a stoke, it is useful to encourage the use of the working limbs so that the paralysed limbs can be supported. The affected limbs should be worked passively (that is gently mobilised by a carer) to prevent contractures.

## Heart disease

Exercise should be of benefit, but should be used within the limits imposed by the client's condition. Medical advice must be sought.

## Lack of motivation

Lack of motivation can be a real problem among some older people. However, it may be possible to encourage movement to old-time music with which they might be familiar. This also becomes part of reminiscence therapy, using stimuli from the past to help clients who may be disoriented or confused.

Even if an older person is unable to move around very much, some exercise is still possible. Even when sitting down, some movement should be of benefit. The session could begin with deep breathing exercises, joint mobility exercises could follow (move fingers, wrists, elbows, shoulders, toes, ankles, knees; whatever is comfortably and safely possible). Some gentle stretching exercises could then complete the session.

It is important to take into consideration the dignity of the client and their individual rights. They must be consulted about possible exercise activity, and their wishes respected.

## Activity 5.10

Devise an exercise programme for a selected client, using the above guidelines. If you are unable to gain access to a client, use a case history, or simply devise some general sets of guidelines for a specific client group, such as people who have lower-body mobility impairment.

**Care point**

Caution should be taken when a client begins a programme of exercise, particularly if they have not exercised for a long time. It is advisable to seek medical advice if there is any doubt. Exercise can benefit many people who have particular care needs, and can be adapted so that most can enjoy some sort of sporting activity.

## Twenty questions

1  Name one risk factor that may be linked with reduced physical activity in children.

2  Name one possible advantage of regular exercise for the older person.

3  Name the three types of muscle in the body.

4  What are bundles of muscle fibres called?

5  Which word describes a situation in which oxygen is not required?

6  Which system subsequently allows energy to be produced very rapidly to meet the requirements of intensive muscular effort?

7  Which muscle fibre type would you expect a marathon runner to have in higher proportion in the leg muscles?

8  Identify one adaptation that occurs as a result of strength training.

9  Name the three main components of blood

10  Which site on the body is usually used for recording the pulse rate?

11  Outline the main difference between arteries and veins.

12  Which substance accumulates in the blood as a result of increased exercise intensity?

13  Identify one adaptation that occurs within the the cardio-vascular system as a result of aerobic exercise taken over a period of time.

14  Briefly explain the difference between internal and external respiration.

15  Name the small structures situated at the end of the bronchioles in the lungs, and identify the process that occurs in them.

16  Outline the physical processes in the body that bring about inspiration.

17  What is the benefit of improving the condition and efficiency of breathing muscles through exercise?

18 Explain the term *residual volume*.

19 Which term describes the tidal volume plus the inspiratory and expiratory reserve volumes?

20 Why are slower, deeper breaths more efficient?

# Quick concepts

| | |
|---|---|
| **Adenosine phosphate** | The immediate source of energy in the muscle |
| **Aerobic** | Requiring the presence of oxygen (cf anaerobic) |
| **Alveoli** | Tiny air sacs in the lungs where oxygen and carbon dioxide exchange takes place |
| **Anaerobic** | Not requiring the presence of oxygen |
| **Concentric contraction** | The muscle shortens and thickens |
| **Diffusion** | The passing of substances through a membrane from a higher to a lower concentration |
| **Eccentric contraction** | Opposite to concentric; the muscle returns to its resting position, but still under resistance (e.g. when lowering a barbell) |
| **Expiration** | Breathing out brought about by elastic recoil of the muscles associated with breathing |
| **External respiration** | The means by which oxygen is obtained from the environment and carbon dioxide released into it |
| **Fasciculi** | Bundles of muscle fibres, many of which, wrapped in a sheet of areolar tissue, make up a muscle |
| **Fast twitch muscle fibre types** | Muscle fibres which contract quickly, producing more force, but which tire quickly |
| **Inspiration** | Breathing in brought about by contraction of the muscles associated with breathing |
| **Inspiratory capacity** | The amount of air that can be inspired with the maximum effort |
| **Internal respiration** | The chain of chemical processes which take place in every cell to free energy |
| **Isometric contraction** | The muscle develops tension. There is no movement of the joint axis |
| **Isotonic contraction** | The muscle develops tension to overcome a resistance, with associated movement of a body part |
| **Lactic acid** | A by-product of anaerobic activity that transports energy from muscle to muscle |
| **Mitochondria** | Specialised structures within the cells in which an aerobic metabolism process takes place |
| **Myoglobin** | A protein material in the muscle that has a strong affinity for oxygen |
| **Pulse** | A wave that travels down the artery following each contraction of the heart |

| | |
|---|---|
| **Residual volume** | The portion of lung capacity that cannot be used |
| **Skeletal muscle** | Controlled by the voluntary part of the nervous system, composed of striated (striped) cells bound together by connective tissue |
| **Slow twitch muscle fibre types** | Muscle fibres which contract and relax slowly but are resistant to fatigue |
| **Stroke volume** | Volume of blood pumped from a ventricle during each contraction of the heart |
| **Target training zone** | The heart rate zone during which exercise is likely to produce the desired effect |
| **Tidal volume** | The amount of air which passes into and out of the lungs during each cycle of quiet breathing |
| **Vital capacity** | Tidal volume plus inspiratory and expiratory reserve volumes |

# Supplementary reading

Hazeldine, R, *Fitness for Sport*, The Crowood Press, 1991

Rowett, H G Q, *Basic Anatomy and Physiology*, John Murray, 1987

Sharkey, B J, *Physiology of Fitness*, Human Kinetics Books, 1990

Wilson, K J W, *Anatomy and Physiology*, Churchill Livingstone, 1987

Wirhed, R, *Athletic Ability and the Anatomy of Motion*, Wolfe Medical Publications Limited, 1991.

# 6 Environmental health provision

## What is covered in this chapter

- Environmental health: the framework of legislation
- Inspection and enforcement agencies
- Social and economic influences

## Introduction

In 1977 the World Health Assembly established a policy *Health for All by the Year 2000*. This policy indicated the environment as a major determinant of human health. It highlighted the need for The World Health Organisation to extend its efforts beyond the traditional curative and preventative medical programmes to a broader approach: to emphasise primary health care, man's environment and its relationship to man's health.

A more recent publication has been the Government White Paper *The Health of the Nation*. This offered significant comment on environmental influences on health.

## Environmental health: the framework of legislation
### The European influence

The framework of legislation to maintain environmental health is influenced by European Union policy. The environment policy, based in the Community Treaty, is now an integral part of the other EU policies. The European Union is the only major international organisation which has an effective legislative and administrative framework and legal capacity in the field of environment.

The relevance of the European framework is that many of our environmental issues have become of global concern. In order to have effective environmental policy, there must be international negotiations on issues such as the ozone layer.

### Environmental pollution

#### Sources of emission
Each year some 500 chemical compounds are put onto the market to add to the 27 000 already in use. The main sources of emissions are:
- domestic and industrial heating and generators
- industrial effluents
- motor vehicles, ships and planes using petroleum or inorganic oil fuels
- industrial products
- agricultural chemicals
- household and domestic products, such as solvents, detergents, paint, varnish, insecticides, medicines, cosmetics, plastic packaging and detergent.

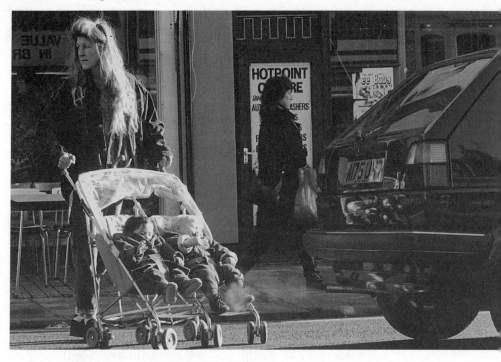

*Cars are among the main sources of environmental pollution*

### Factors influencing the distribution of pollutants

After entering the physical environment, pollutants are subjected to a whole range of factors liable to influence their distribution. Various meteorological conditions, such as wind, rain, fog or temperature inversions, play a part. Pollutants can be transformed, giving rise to new compounds: for example, photochemical reactions due to solar radiation cause the formation of irritant and phytotoxic peracyl nitrates (an element of smog) from components of car exhaust and aeroplane reactors.

### Harmful effects of environmental pollution

Acid rain, caused by a mixture of air pollutants, has caused the death of whole forests; fish have disappeared from thousands of lakes in Scandinavia. Declining numbers of acid-sensitive plant and animal species have been recorded in many countries, including the UK.

### The Montreal Protocol

The Montreal Protocol was signed in September 1987 in order to limit emissions of the CFC family of chemicals (chlorofluorocarbons) which are damaging the ozone layer. This was the first truly global agreement on protection of the environment. It was also the first global pre-emptive environmental agreement: it looks ahead to face a distant threat and enables action to be taken now to prevent grave damage in the future. It also set a precedent for further global action against threats to the environment.

### The ozone layer

Life on earth depends upon ozone because ozone acts as a sponge, absorbing ultraviolet radiation from the sun and shielding the earth from the most harmful radiation. Radiation causes skin cancer and eye damage. Increased levels would affect the climate and damage human health as well as plants and marine life. The wider environmental effects of ozone depletion include reduced crop growth and damage to marine life.

### The indoor environment

The quality of the indoor environment may have implications for some individuals. Asthma, for example, may be exacerbated by indoor pollution caused primarily by tobacco smoke. The increasing practice of creating smoke-free zones within the workplace and in many public areas is a response to a growing awareness of the dangers of passive smoking.

## Water quality

### Contaminated tap water

It is stated in *The Health of the Nation* that supplies that do not comply with the European Community Drinking Water Directive are not necessarily a danger to health. However, 20 per cent of people suffering from contamination of tap water from the parasite cryptosporidium require hospital treatment. A study conducted in America in 1991 concluded that 31 per cent of reported gastrointestinal illnesses were water-related and preventable.

### Contaminated groundwater

There does not appear to be a commitment to protecting Britain's aquifers (a significant body of groundwater) from contamination by toxic seepage from waste dumps or landfill sites. Aquifers provide half the total drinking water and one fifth of the country's total water requirement.

### The increasing incidence of water pollution

More than twice as many water pollution incidents were reported to the National Rivers Authority (the NRA – the government body responsible for protecting the water environment in England and Wales) in 1989–90 as in 1980–1, which reflects the growing problem of river pollution. Since 1985, 15 per cent of the total length of rivers have declined in quality.

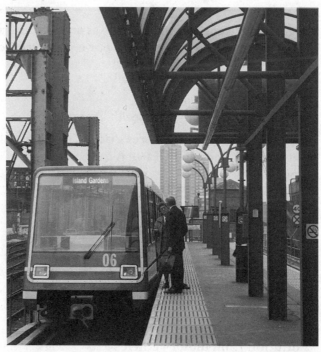

*Docklands Light Railway, London: many public areas are becoming no-smoking zones*

### Pesticides

The European Directive (80/778/EEC) specifies the maximum admissible concentration of pesticides in drinking water. However, the Friends of the Earth found in 1988 that 298 water supplies exceeded the specified amount for any single pesticide. Breaches of the maximum admissible concentration for total pesticides were recorded on 76 occasions.

In the years 1992–4 there has been evidence of high levels of the pesticide dieldrin discharged into the River Severn. Although dieldrin is banned in all EU countries under directive 79/117/EEC, it is present in animal fleeces imported from the third world.

### Bathing waters

In 1991, 24 per cent of UK bathing waters that were tested failed to meet the minimum required European standards for bacteria in bathing water. Only waters that have been officially designated as bathing water have to comply with the European standards. As no inland waters have been designated in the UK, there is no guarantee of water purity for people who swim in rivers and lakes.

### Lead in drinking water

One of the most recent concerns has been about the levels of lead in drinking water. Lead is dissolved into drinking water from lead supply pipes. Lead is a poisonous metal which interferes with enzymes essential to the working of almost every part of the body. Links have been found between lead in blood and damage to kidneys, the reproductive system and vitamin D formation. Lead has also been classified as a possible cause of cancer.

Over 4 million homes in England may be supplied with water where lead concentrations exceed the World Health Organisation guideline of 10 micrograms per litre.

## Activity 6.1

Find out the steps that you can take as an individual, a family or as a group at work, school or college in order to help prevent and reduce water pollution. Sources of information include:

- The Friends of the Earth
- your local NRA office
- your local Environmental Health Directorate.

Identify the particular measures that you can take to help reduce lead in drinking water. The Friends of the Earth is the best source of information for this particular aspect of water pollution.

## Air quality

### The need for clean air

Air is the most essential element to sustain life. Every single day, from birth to death a person absorbs about twelve cubic metres of air. Any adulteration of its purity is, therefore, of primary importance. Sufficiently small particles can penetrate to the pulmonary alveoli where they can produce harmful effects, and can also pass into the circulatory system.

### Pollution from motor vehicles

In the winter of 1952, a combination of high emissions of sulphur dioxide and particulates from coal burning gave rise to *smog*, which led to an estimated 4 000 deaths in London over a period of a month. The threat today originates from motor vehicles, which produce more air pollution than any other source. Other emissions of nitrogen dioxide, sulphur and carbon are known to be respiratory irritants. The World Health Organisation's guidelines for nitrogen dioxide levels are exceeded on the roads in Britain. Although the increased use of catalytic converters will reduce the levels of pollutants, the growth in the volume of traffic may negate this reduction. *The Health of the Nation* demands a reduction in nitrogen dioxide of 50 per cent by the year 2000.

### Legal action towards cleaner air

A variety of industrial and commercial emissions give rise to complaints which are investigated by the Environmental Health Directorate. If there is no improvement following informal action, statutory action and possible prosecution of offenders may follow. Some major nuisances are woodworking machinery, paint spraying, chemical processes and extractor systems on catering premises.

The Smoke Control Area programmes of the 1960s attempted to limit domestic emissions with the widespread replacement of raw coal by oil, gas and solid smokeless fuels. This dramatically reduced the large amount of pollution from domestic fuel burning.

Garden bonfires and the burning of waste from industrial and commercial activities such as scrap yards and stubble burning are subject to control. Where a statutory nuisance can be proved, legal action can be taken.

**Activity 6.2**

Air quality is monitored through a number of permanent monitoring sites which form part of the national network set up to comply with the European Commission Directive on standards for air quality. In particular, they monitor smoke, particulates, sulphur dioxide and nitrous oxide. Find out (from your local Environmental Health Directorate) if there are any of these sites in your local authority area; if not, find out where information on local air quality is available.

**Activity 6.3**

As for Activity 6.1 on water, find out how you, as an individual, a family or a group at work, school or college can contribute towards the reduction of air pollution. Again the best source of information is The Friends of the Earth.

**Activity 6.4**

Obtain the briefing sheet *Air Quality* from The Friends of the Earth (1990). Study the enclosed table which provides information on different pollutants and their sources, the effects upon health and the environment, air quality standards and the UK levels of these pollutants. Write an essay comparing and contrasting the relationships of the different pollutants with these variables, or simplify the findings into the form of a teaching session to be directed towards colleagues or your fellow students.

## Noise pollution

Excessive, unwanted noise is one of the great problems of modern life. As well as being annoying, it can cause ill-health and stress. Noise can be broadly divided into three types:

- domestic noise (for example, arguments, televisions and radios, dogs barking)

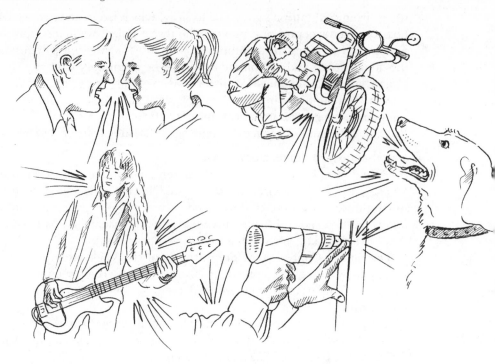

*Domestic noise is one of the hazards of modern life*

- industrial noise
- entertainment noise.

Legislative action can be most effectively applied to entertainment noise, as mar establishments such as clubs, discos and public houses require public entertainmer licences and planning permission. The local council can impose conditions on the us of such premises with the aim of preventing noise-nuisance.

### Activity 6.5

It is possible for a person who is aggrieved by a noise nuisance to take a private action. Find out how this can be done. Try your local library, Citizens Advice Burea or Law Centre for information. Does your local Environmental Health Directorate provide specific information on this issue?

### Activity 6.6

List the sources of noise within your working environment or work experience placement. Give each item a rating of between 1 and 10 according to how loud and intrusive you think the noise is. If feasible, gain the opinions of clients or colleagues as to the noise levels of their immediate environment. Are there any ways in which noise can be reduced in their environment?

## Food hygiene and the sale of food

### The Food Safety Act (1990)

The Food Safety Act (1990) replaced the Act of 1984. Within the Act, food includ such items as:

- drink

- articles and substances of no nutritional value which are used for human consumption
- chewing gum and similar products
- substances which are used as ingredients in the preparation of food.

It does not include such things as live animals or live fish.

The Act defines such activities as 'rendering food injurious to health', 'selling food not complying with food safety requirements' and provides for the inspection and seizure of suspected food. It allows for improvement notices and prohibition orders to be served where appropriate, and includes emergency prohibition notices and orders.

### Consumer protection

Consumer protection is promoted by reference to the illegality of selling substandard food, and of falsely describing or presenting food.

Premises that are used for the purpose of a food business should be registered and licensed. Public analysts have been appointed for the purpose of examining samples of suspected food. The Act makes provision for the activities of these individuals, including access to premises.

### The Food Hygiene (General) Regulations (1970)

The regulations of 1970 cover such subjects as the repair and condition of food rooms, cleanliness, the personal hygiene of staff, washing facilities, lighting, ventilation and temperature control.

Where contraventions of the legislation are found, an informal notice is served on the person carrying on the business, listing matters which require attention. If the work is not carried out within a reasonable period of time, the Environmental Health Officer will recommend the instigation of legal proceedings. For each contravention of the 1970 Regulations, a fine of up to £2000 may be imposed by the Magistrates' Court and imprisonment of the proprietor or closure of the premises may result for serious offences.

## Housing and building regulations

### The role of local authorities

Local authorities have a duty under the Public Health and Housing Acts to review housing conditions in their areas in order to detect conditions which may be prejudicial to health and to identify unfit or unsatisfactory housing.

In houses where conditions prejudicial to health are found, the council serves a statutory notice on the owner, requiring him to carry our work to put matters right. If he fails to do so, the council may carry out the work and charge him with costs, or take him to court where the magistrates may make an order requiring him to do whatever is necessary to rectify conditions.

Where unsatisfactory conditions are found which render a house unfit to live in, or where improvements are necessary to bring them up to modern standards, a council may adopt one of two approaches:

- a notice may be served on the owner requiring him to repair the house if it can be done at reasonable cost.
- if the house cannot be made fit at reasonable cost a closing order or demolition order may be made.

### Houses in multiple occupation

'Houses in multiple occupation' are those occupied by people who do not form a single household. Housing conditions may be unsatisfactory and unsafe due to inadequate sanitary facilities, unsatisfactory cooking arrangements, overcrowding and fire hazards. These houses are often occupied by some of the most vulnerable members of the community. The council has the power to serve statutory notices to improve and control physical conditions in these properties as well as standards of management.

## Local building policies

Local building policies aim to secure the health, safety, welfare and convenience of people in or about buildings, and to further the conservation of fuel and power, by promoting adherence to building regulations and allied legislation. The scope of building control includes:

- structural stability
- fire engineering
- site preparation
- resistance to damp
- toxic substances
- sound insulation
- ventilation
- hygiene
- drainage and waste disposal
- heating appliances
- stairways
- conservation of fuel
- access for the disabled
- short-lived material.

Building control regulations also apply to the inspection of dangerous structures and to demolitions.

# Health and safety at work

### The duty of the employer towards employees

The Health and Safety at Work Act (1974) states that it is the duty of every employer to ensure, as far as is reasonably practicable, the health, safety and welfare at work of all his or her employees. Provision and maintenance of plant and systems of work must be made that are, as far as is reasonably practicable, safe and without risks to health.

Similar provisions apply to the use, handling, storage and transport of articles and substances and cover all items used at work and all work activities. Other requirements cover:

- the provision of instruction, training and supervision
- the maintenance of workplaces and means of entry and exit
- the adequacy of facilities and arrangements for welfare
- the need to provide a written statement of safety policy for the attention of all employees

There is a requirement to have employee safety representatives and safety committees.

### Obligations towards non-employees

Under the Health and Safety at Work Act, there are also obligations to members of the public, as well as to the employees of sub-contractors, etc. who work on an employer's premises. The terms of the Act are very broad in an attempt to cover most

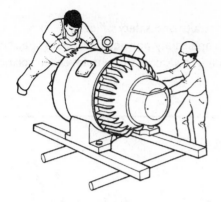
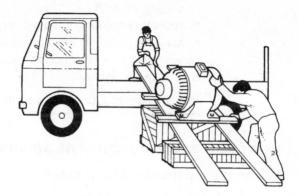

*There are regulations governing such areas as moving heavy loads or hazardous substances*

people and most circumstances. There are further extensive responsibilities for manufacturers, suppliers and installers of plant equipment, substances, etc. to ensure that their products are designed and installed safely.

### Standards

The words 'as far as is reasonably practicable' appear throughout the Act, as it is difficult to prescribe the exact standard of acceptable risk to health and safety in widely differing workplaces. The Health and Safety at Work Act did not replace existing legislation, so that there are a number of acts, such as The Factories Act, The Office Shop and Railway Premises Act and The Shop Act, which give more detailed standards. In addition there are a large number of safety regulations which give more precise specifications on particular health hazards (for example, asbestos, lead), machinery hazards and on particular industries. A third source of guidance is the various Codes of Practice. They do not have the force of law, but they can be used by health and safety inspectors to influence employers.

### The responsibilities of employees

The Act also places obligations on all individual employees to co-operate with an employer to carry out his duties, to take 'reasonable care for the health and safety of himself and other persons' and not to 'intentionally or recklessly interfere with or misuse anything provided in the interests of health, safety or welfare'.

> It is difficult for legislation to prescribe the exact standard of acceptable risk to health and safety, but care workers need to recognise and avoid the numerous
> *Care point* > potential hazards to both staff and patients or clients that exist within hospitals and other caring establishments. The Control of Substances Hazardous to Health (COSHH, 1988) regulations is one piece of legislation designed to protect staff and others, for example patients or clients.

### Activity 6.7

How effective is the application of the Health and Safety at Work Act in your place of work (or your work experience placement)?

Devise a checklist that includes such items as:

• availability of a health and safety policy

- training for staff
- general awareness of the identity of the health and safety officer
- availability and implementation of health and safety policies that relate specifically to your area of work, such as manual handling, awareness of employees in relation to their responsibilities.

Which additional items can you think of?

# Inspection and enforcement agencies

## Environmental health directorates

Environmental Health Directorates are responsible for advising on a wide range of topics and for enforcing regulations at a local level. Directorate staff include Environmental Health Officers, Authorised Meat Inspectors and Building Control Officers.

## Environmental Health Officers

### Controlling noise

Noise control is an important function of the Environmental Health Directorate. If informal action fails to resolve the problem, proceedings may be instituted. The Environmental Health Officer must satisfy the Local Health Authority that a noise nuisance exists or is likely to recur. A statutory notice is served on the person causing the nuisance; he or she may appeal against it to a magistrates court. If the appeal fails and the nuisance continues, a prosecution is likely to follow. The Environmental Health Officers contribute to the planning and developmental control processes by providing information about existing and proposed noise levels to the Directorate of Planning. They also give advice on suitable control measures.

### Drinking water

Environmental Health Officers undertake regular sampling of drinking water supplies for chemical and bacteriological examination. This is particularly important for private water supplies from wells and bore holes. The bacteriological and chemical quality of swimming pool water is regularly monitored. The officers give advice when water quality is unsatisfactory and retesting takes place to ensure that the advice is effective.

### Monitoring food hygiene

Another function of The Environmental Health Directorate is the inspection and examination of food supplies. This involves general surveillance of food production facilities, storage and retail premises. These premises are visited regularly in order to ensure that they comply with the relevant legislation.

EHOs are also involved in the investigation of food complaints. Problems with food can arise during the production, transportation, storage and retail stages. Prosecutions may be taken under the provisions of the Food Safety Act (1990).

Unfit or spoiled foodstuffs may be condemned either following a routine inspection or on receipt of a complaint. An Environmental Health Officer will examine the food and if necessary it can be 'seized'. Subsequent legal action can secure its destruction.

At local levels, sampling programmes ensure that all types of food are subjected to examination by the Public Analyst, and that producers are complying with legally specified compositional and labelling standards.

# Authorised meat inspectors

The Environmental Health Directorate is also responsible for enforcing the legislation governing the slaughter of animals intended for human consumption.

Authorised meat inspectors often have permanent posts within abattoirs to check that the EU requirements for animal welfare, suitability for human consumption and cleanliness are met. A considerable amount of meat is rejected as being unfit for human consumption.

# Building control officers

Building control officers ensure that all new building work satisfies the requirements of the building regulations and allied legislation. They carry out site inspections to check that building works are carried out to the required standard.

# The National Rivers Authority

The NRA (see page 97) is responsible for licensing all discharges to rivers and for ensuring that environmental protection standards are met.

# The enforcement of health and safety legislation

There are three main steps that can be taken to compel an employer to provide and maintain a safe and healthy place of work:
- improvement notices
- prohibition notices
- fines or threats of imprisonment.

The health and safety executive inspectors have the power to inspect premises and to issue notices. The executive is also a source of advice and information and can refer to the Employment Medical Advisory Service.

# Activity 6.8

Visit your local district council offices, and ask for information about local environmental health provision. How easy is it to find the information?
Alternatively, make enquiries by telephone, asking for written information to be sent to you. Is the information presented clearly? Visit your local library and find out if written material is available there about the local Environmental Health Directorate.

We have seen how *The Health of the Nation* recognises environmental influences on health. There is a view that professionals working in health care should adopt a leading role in pressurising influential agencies to take concrete measures to protect the environment. The Royal College of Nursing has established an environmental working party in recognition of growing concern about pollution of the environment and the effects on health.

# Activity 6.9

Consider the possible environmental effects on the health of a client group in your work experience placement, if this is appropriate. Using one client (change the name to protect their privacy), draw a mind map (a diagram with the client in the centre of the page and arrows pointing towards them to indicate environmental influences on their health). Aim to be as specific as possible in relation to this individual person. You could refer to the section on noise (Activity 6.5) for one possible example. If you do not currently have contact with clients, then carry out this exercise with an imaginary client.

| Care point | Carers should be familiar with environmental determinants of health: they will then be more effective in meeting the health needs of their client group. |

# Social and economic influences

## Pressure groups

Legislative change has been necessary to protect the environment. However, this has often been instigated and informed by pressure from such bodies as the World Health Organisation and The Friends of the Earth (FoE). Organisations such as FoE and Greenpeace also work to increase public awareness about environmental issues. By mobilising public opinion, they aim to persuade politicians and industry to take action at international, national and local levels.

## Media involvement

In some instances celebrities have given ecological issues a high profile – Sting, for example has highlighted the destruction of the rainforests; The Prince of Wales has drawn attention to the need for attractive modern architecture. When this happens, remedial and preventative action has to be seen to be taken.

## Individual responsibility

People are being encouraged to take individual responsibility for the protection of the environment. The provision of bottle, can, paper and clothing banks for recycling household waste are examples of how this individual responsibility is promoted. At times the Government has been accused in various sections of the media of taking insufficient action to maintain the environment.

## Children and young people

Children and young people are increasingly being made aware about environmental issues, in schools as well as on television and in magazines. It is increasingly likely that an informed generation will grow up applying their heightened awareness to their own practices and it is hoped that they will also keep up the pressure on governments and industry to take measures to look after the environment.

## The economy

The economy and energy consumption are closely linked. Energy production underpins the development of industrial economies. However, the deployment of massive quantities of energy poses ecological problems of the same scale. There is often a conflict between economists and ecologists, between profit-making and maintaining the environment. Industries could, however, work together to benefit both themselves and the environment. The report of the World Commission on Environment and

Development to the UN in 1987 and the Earth Summit in Rio de Janeiro in 1992 have challenged human economic activities that have previously been more concerned with profit than sustainability.

## Recycling

Recycling is a key component in achieving a more harmonious relationship between industry and ecology. The ideal to work towards is the creation of industrial parks that function as ecosystems.

## Economic influences

Economic influences may affect general awareness of environmental health issues. This can be seen in the disproportionate amount of funding allocated to various aspects of health education. Health education departments have been criticised for not paying enough attention to such issues as river or coastal pollution, or damp housing. The general public needs as much information about the health risks associated with these as about excessive smoking and alcohol abuse.

## Twenty questions

1 How does an emphasis on environmental health differ from a traditional, medically orientated approach?

2 Name the 1992 Government White Paper which made significant comments about environmental influences on health.

3 Which policy influences the framework of legislation that maintains environmental health?

4 Why is the European framework relevant to issues affecting our environment?

5 Which act replaced the Food Act (1984)?

6 Which people are appointed for the purpose of examining samples of suspected food?

7 Which acts impose a duty on the local authority to review housing conditions?

8 Name one approach that a local council may take if they find conditions which make a house unfit to live in.

9 In 'houses of multiple occupation', which aspects may be subject to scrutiny?

10 What do local building policies hope to achieve?

11 What are the three main categories of noise pollution?

12 Name two main sources of emissions that contribute to environmental pollution.

13 Name one factor that influences the distribution of pollutants.

14 Name one harmful effect of environmental pollution.

15 Give one reason why life on earth depends upon ozone.

16 What is a major factor affecting the quality of the indoor environment?

17 What is the greatest source of air pollution?

18 Which individual has the power to inspect premises and issue notices in checking health and safety?

19 Name one possible function of an Environmental Health Officer.

20 In one sentence, outline a conflict between economics and ecology.

## Supplementary reading

The Department of Health,*The Health of the Nation*, HMSO, 1992

Krieps, R (ed.), *Environment and Health: A Holistic Approach*, Avebury, 1989

*Air Quality* Briefing Sheet, Friends of the Earth, 1990

Lees, A and McVeigh, K, *An investigation of Pesticide Pollution in Drinking Water in England and Wales,* Friends of the Earth, 1988

Purdom, P W, *Environmental Health, Second Edition,* Academic Press, 1980

Rowland, A J and Cooper, P, *Environment and Health*, Edward Arnold, 1983

Stranks J, *The handbook of Health and Safety in Practice*, Pitman, 1986

*Water* (leaflet), Friends of the Earth, 1992

*Air pollution* (leaflet), Friends of the Earth, 1991

The Friends of the Earth provide a variety of reading materials: leaflets, booklets, briefings, reports, magazines, manuals and books on a range of environmental issues.

A useful journal for information and discussion on the issues raised in this chapter is the *New Scientist*, published weekly by IPC Magazines Ltd.

# 7 Monitoring human body processes

## What is covered in this chapter

- The role of pathological services
- The role of physiological measurement
- Imaging techniques
- Bioelectric events: the electrocardiogram
- Blood tests for prevention and diagnosis
- The microscopic study of cells
- Identification of bacteria and viruses
- Screening services

## Introduction

It is not always possible to tell if the body is healthy just by looking at a person, or even for a doctor always to diagnose ill health by examining a patient. To help diagnosis and to attempt to detect disease at an early stage there are ways of monitoring body processes. Some investigations are very simple and non-invasive – they do not cause the client any distress; yet they may detect and allow treatment of potentially lethal diseases. One example is the measurement of blood pressure. Raised blood pressure (hypertension), is known as 'the silent killer'. It may not give rise to any symptoms but silently damages the body's blood vessels. 30 per cent of those over fifty years old in Britain have hypertension. By checking everyone's blood pressure this condition can be detected and treated at an early stage.

Monitoring of body processes may need the facilities provided in hospital if the investigation is complex. An **angiogram**, for example involves injecting dye into the blood vessels to show any abnormalities; this has to be done in hospital. Other investigations involve a visit to the hospital laboratory, for example to have a blood sample taken, but other tests may be done in the person's home or even by the client themselves, for example testing urine for abnormalities that may detect diabetes. A very simple monitoring that can be done at home is checking body weight to keep this in control and prevent obesity.

There are many ways of monitoring body processes: these include physiological measurements such as recording the electrical activity of the heart and tests of respiratory function. There are also imaging techniques such as radiology and ultrasound that give a picture of the internal organs of the body. All these tests are interrelated and good communication between the services concerned is essential for early diagnosis and the sharing of information to benefit the patient.

## Reasons for investigation

Reasons for investigation might include:
- part of a medical examination for a new job (a career in nursing or the armed

forces, for example, requires certain blood tests as part of the individual's health profile)
- screening in an attempt to detect disease
- to help doctors in the diagnosis of medical conditions (or before undergoing an operation)
- to follow the progress of a disorder.

Prevention of disease is always better than cure and the emphasis in the health service is now towards remaining healthy rather than treating disease. The government publication *The Health of the Nation* emphasises the importance of health education in the prevention of disease and the early detection of possible causes of ill health. Screening services such as cervical screening and mammography for early detection of breast cancer work towards this aim. Some of the screening services provided for the public are discussed at the end of this chapter.

## The role of pathological services

**Pathology** is the study of disease which is achieved by observing samples of blood, urine, faeces and diseased tissue. The pathology laboratory in a hospital has several departments:
- **microbiology**
- **haematology**
- **biochemistry**

## The microbiology laboratory

If a specimen is sent to the laboratory they will firstly check to see if the bacteria can be seen under the microscope with staining. They will then culture the specimen in special nutrient gel over a period of 48 hours to see if it is contaminated with bacteria; if it is, the bacteria will grow rapidly. If the bacteria do grow, the laboratory will test their response to common antibiotics, and will send a report to the doctor with the recommended drugs, so that the doctor may treat the infection in the most efficient way. Ideally the samples should be collected before the patient starts on any antibiotic treatment.

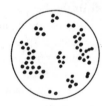

*A culture plate showing staphylococci*

### Urine specimens

Specimens of urine are normally best taken in the morning when the urine is more concentrated. Urine is normally sterile – it does not have any bacteria in it. If bacteria do grow in a urine culture, there is a urinary tract infection which will need treatment to prevent the infection spreading to the kidneys.

One of the commonest organisms to infect urine is eserichia coli, which comes from the bowel. The presence of the organism makes the urine smell of fish.

Great care has to be taken to ensure that a urine specimen is not contaminated when it is collected. To try to prevent contamination a mid-stream urine specimen is taken. The client should be clean (after a bath would be a good time), and start the flow of urine into the toilet. The middle amount of urine is caught in a sterile jug and the client finishes passing urine in the toilet. The urine in the jug is now carefully poured into a sterile container from the laboratory and labelled with the client's name and details. Urine specimens should reach the laboratory within one hour or be refrigerated at 40 °C.

### Blood specimens

A specimen of blood to be cultivated is called a blood culture and has to be put into special bottles with nutrient fluid already in them. This sample is taken when an infection in the blood is suspected. The samples have to go to the laboratory immediately, where they are incubated (kept at a constant warm temperature). The bacteria are most likely to be present when the temperature is raised, so a specimen is usually taken when the temperature is at its highest. If bacteria are multiplying in the bloodstream this is septicaemia, which may be life threatening.

### Sputum specimens

Sputum is never free from bacteria. Those that are always present are called the normal flora and are not harmful. A specimen is taken in order to detect a chest infection. It is necessary to ensure that the client does actually give a specimen of sputum, obtained from the lungs by coughing, and does not just spit saliva into the container.

If tuberculosis is suspected, this culture has to be specially requested and the bacteria stained with a particular dye. Application of acid would normally remove this dye, but the tubercle bacillus is dye-fast even in the presence of acid. For this reason it is called an **acid-fast bacillus**.

### Faeces

Samples of faeces are needed if the client has diarrhoea and an infection is possible. The microbiologist is looking for such organisms as salmonella typhi or shigella in the faeces. When faeces are collected there should be no urine or toilet paper in the sample.

### Nose and throat swabs

A throat swab is ordered to detect the presence of bacteria in the throat. It is ordered when the client has a sore throat accompanied by the signs and symptoms of a bacterial infection. The swabs come in sterile tubes and have to be carefully used so that contamination does not occur. The throat swab has to reach the back of the throat without touching the tongue or mouth.

Nose swabs are taken for suspected infection which may be symptomless. This may be done routinely on some hospital wards to ensure that staff are not harbouring harmful bacteria in their nose that could be passed on to patients. One such bacteria that can be carried in this way is the multi-resistant staphylococcus aureus, so called because it is resistant to so many antibiotics. Although harmless in the healthy when living in the nose or on the skin, it can be very dangerous if it gets into wounds, say on a surgical ward.

### Wound swabs

If a wound becomes inflamed and perhaps produces pus, a swab is taken so that the responsible organism can be identified and treated.

### Cerebrospinal fluid

Cerebrospinal fluid surrounds the brain and spinal cord. A sample is removed in a procedure called a lumbar puncture. If organisms are present the patient has meningitis. Cerebrospinal fluid is usually clear but if bacteria are present it is cloudy.

## The haematology laboratory

Investigations in the haematology laboratory relate to the production of blood cells, their functions and diseases which affect them.

In a test called a bone marrow puncture, a sample to measure the production of blood cells is taken from the bone marrow (the site of cell manufacture). The bone most commonly used is the sternum (chest bone). A special marrow puncture needle with a syringe aspirates, or draws out, the sample.

Maturity and function of blood cells may be checked by this test. This helps to confirm diagnosis of anaemia, a condition in which there is a reduction in the number of red blood cells or of the pigment within them. This reduction means that the red cells are less able to transport oxygen around the body.

## The biochemistry laboratory

The main fluid analysed in the biochemistry laboratory is blood. The most frequent investigation is the measurement of the levels of the different electrolytes in the blood. These include sodium, potassium and chlorine. The levels of these substances change rapidly in cases of dehydration or any imbalance of the body. This is probably the most common investigation that the doctor does. The biochemistry laboratory also estimates the level of urea in the blood. This test identifies whether the kidneys are functioning adequately. Urea is the breakdown product of proteins; if the kidneys cannot excrete well, the level of urea in the blood will rise (The function of the kidneys was explained in detail in Chapter 2).

### Serology

**Serology** is the study of blood serum and its constituents. Serological studies are necessary when, for instance, defining a person's blood group. This procedure is described later in the chapter. The blood used for these samples is venous blood and is easily obtained from a superficial vein by **phlebotomy**, although the procedure is more difficult in children and the elderly. The elderly often have very visible veins which are nevertheless hard and difficult for the needle of the phlebotomist to enter.

Serum is also studied to detect the presence of such diseases as viral hepatitis. In this case the laboratory is looking for the presence of antibodies and antigens in the blood.

### Histology

Histology, the study of tissues under the microscope using staining techniques, is discussed in the section *The microscopic study of cells*, on page 121.

### Immunological status

A blood sample is needed to establish **immunological status**, that is enabling the doctor to identify which diseases the client has already met and recovered from; antibodies to these diseases will be detected in the blood. Not only infections can be investigated in this way, but also certain diseases where there is a disordered immune system. One such disease is rheumatoid arthritis; in this case the laboratory is looking for the rheumatoid factor, an antibody, which is diagnostic of rheumatoid arthritis.

# The role of physiological measurement

## Audiogram

An **audiogram** is a graphic record of a hearing test which is carried out using specialised equipment called an audiometer. This measures hearing of sound at different frequencies and can be used to help diagnose deafness.

## Respiratory measurement

The measurement of air taken into and expelled from the lungs is **spirometry**. Changes in lung volumes provide the best measurement of obstruction to airflow in the respiratory passages.

Various measurements are taken of lung capacity. Vital capacity was discussed in Chapter 5, *The respiratory system after exercise*; it is the volume of air breathed out after the client has breathed in as fully as possible. The normal capacity is approximately 2500–3000 millilitres. It is higher in males than females. Vital capacity is reduced in obstructive lung disease such as bronchitis. Forced vital capacity measurements are taken at the bedside in the form of the 'peak flow' measurement. The patient inhales and then forcibly and rapidly exhales into the peak flow machine which registers the amount of air exhaled.

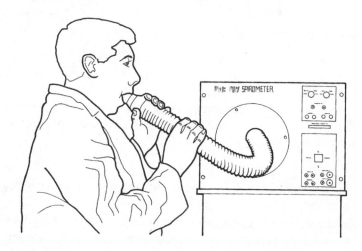

*A spirometer in use*

# Imaging techniques

Imaging techniques are tests that provide a picture of some kind that can be interpreted. There have been great advances in this area in the past twenty years. We can now look at tiny little sections of the brain, for example.

## X-ray studies: radiography

X-rays use electromagnetic radiation of very short wavelength which has great penetrating power in matter that is opaque to light. This means that solid matter shows up well on X-rays. Bones are easily seen and fractures can be detected. On a chest X-ray, the ribs are white and the lungs are almost black. A photograph of a chest X-ray is shown on the following page.

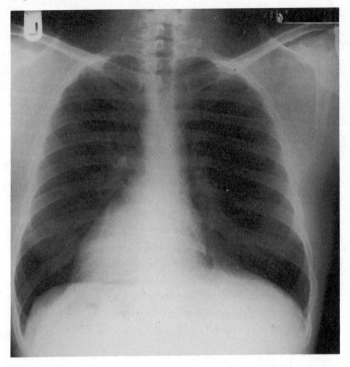

*An X-ray of the chest of a healthy adult*

The chest X-ray is probably one of the most frequently performed. Lung disease suc
as bronchitis can be detected; sometimes lung cancer can be seen. Fluid accumulatio
in the pleura (the coverings of the lungs), an effusion, can be seen. X-rays are bes
performed in the radiography department, but if the client is very ill in hospital,
portable X-ray can be carried out at the bedside. A chest X-ray costs the Nationa
Health Service about £10.

**Care point**

Metal objects should be removed from the patient before X-ray as these obscure
the vision on the X-ray film.
Great care is needed to avoid unnecessary exposure to X-rays as radiation is
harmful in large quantities. Radiographers and those working in the X-ray department have to wear a badge that registers the amount of radiation to which they
have been exposed. This level is checked at weekly intervals to ensure that safety
levels are maintained.

## Computed tomography (CT)

**Computed tomography** enables a complex 3-D picture to be seen. It is built up usin
the computer. This is the type of picture taken in a brain and small tumours or haem
orrhages into the brain can be detected. A CT examination costs £100–200.

### Contrast media

Sometimes radiographs can reveal more if the organ under investigation is first mad
opaque. For example, if a person is to have a stomach X-ray, a barium meal is giver
Barium is a harmless contrast medium which is taken orally. The barium is radic
opaque and makes the outline of the stomach show up clearly on the X-ray. Stomac

ulcers as well as cancer of the stomach can often be identified by this method.

Sometimes radio-opaque dyes are used to show up certain areas or organs. In the investigation of kidney disease, for example, a dye is injected into the vein of the arm. When the dye reaches the kidneys it outlines them on the X-ray and the doctor can tell if one of the kidneys is not working well, or if, for instance, there is a stone in the kidney.

> *Care point* ⊳ Following the X-ray, the client should be encouraged to take fluids to help eliminate the barium. An aperient may be given, as the barium is constipating. The client should be warned that their stools will be chalky white for several days.

### Mammography
**Mammography** is an X-ray examination of the breast. It can detect breast cancer one to two years before a lump may be felt.

### Thermography
Thermography measures the heat produced by parts of the body; the measurements are recorded on photographic paper sensitive to infrared radiation. The picture produced is called a thermogram. Areas of poor circulation in the body produce less heat. A tumour will usually have an increased blood supply and will be seen on the film as a 'hot' spot. The technique is used in the diagnosis of breast cancer.

### Bone scan
A bone scan is often used to detect cancer metastases in bones. After the intravenous injection of radioactive material, the skeleton is examined by a scanning camera.

### Ultrasound
Ultrasound uses high frequencies inaudible to the human ear to produce pictures of body structures. Structures inside the body that are not opaque to X-rays can be seen. Unlike X-rays, the procedure does not subject the client to harmful radiation. Ultrasound is used to see the foetus in the womb and to monitor its development, and also to locate tumours or stones, for example gallstones, inside the body. The vibratory effects of the sound waves can also be used to break up kidney stones. The cost varies between £20–50. It is therefore more expensive than a plain X-ray but less than a CT scan.

### Echocardiography
Echocardiography uses ultrasound techniques to produce a picture of the heart. Valvular abnormalities and congenital defects can be diagnosed. The process is similar to ultrasound: sound waves of very high frequency inaudible to the human ear are used and are bounced back from internal structures to build up pictures similar to X-rays.

# Bioelectric events

## The electrocardiogram (ECG)

Heart tissue is highly specialised and is capable of automatic, rhythmic contraction. The heart beat starts as an electrical impulse at a specific point in the heart, the sino-atrial node. From this point the impulse travels through the conducting system of the heart causing first the atria (upper chambers) to beat and then the ventricles (lower chambers).

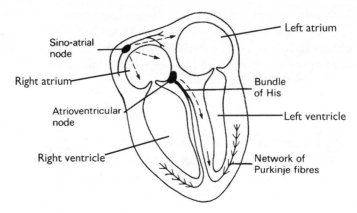

*The conduction system of the heart*

Electrodes applied to the skin can measure the currents produced by the electrical activity in the heart. The electrocardiogram records these electrical impulses in the form of waves on the graph. A normal **electrocardiograph** is shown below.

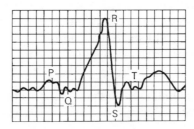

Key
P = Atria contract
QRS = Ventricles contract
T = Heart relaxes

*A normal electrocardiogram tracing*

An electrocardiogram can help to diagnose heart attacks and is a valuable tool for observation of people with heart disease. In many disorders of the heart the electrocardiograph changes in a certain way and this can help the doctor in his diagnosis. If a patient suffers a heart attack or lowered blood supply to the heart, the shape of some of the waves changes. Other abnormalities may occur in infection of the heart or in heart failure when the heart can no longer pump efficiently.

The electrical activity of the heart may be continuously monitored using a cardiac monitor. Electrodes are placed on the client's chest and attached to a monitor at the bedside. The monitor displays the ECG so that any changes can be noted. This is necessary if a client has an irregular beat or disorders of rhythm following a heart attack. These rhythm disturbances could be the first indications of possible problems which might lead to a cardiac arrest. Any changes in the monitor should be reported to the nurse in charge.

**Care point**   A client having an electrocardiograph should be as relaxed as possible, as any movement will alter the tracing. The procedure should be carefully explained so that the client is not nervous, and carers should emphasise the importance of lying still.

# Blood tests for prevention and diagnosis

Investigations of blood are used as a method of screening to ascertain the individual's health status. Blood is the only fluid that comes into contact with all areas of the body and samples are easy to obtain. The composition of blood reflects the function of many bodily activities and the results obtained from blood tests are always compared to a normal body range. The normal ranges are given in the table below.

## Normal blood ranges

| Blood count | Men | Women |
|---|---|---|
| Haemoglobin | 13.5–18 g/dl | 11.5–16.5 g/dl |
| Packed cell volume | 40–54% | 36–47% |

| | Men and women | |
|---|---|---|
| White cell count | $4–11 \times 10^9$ /l | |
| Platelet count | $150–400 \times 10^9$ /l | |

| Biochemistry | |
|---|---|
| Sodium | 135–147 mmol/l |
| Potassium | 3.8–5.0 mmol/l |
| Urea | 2.5–6.5 mmol/l |
| Glucose | 3.4–6.5 mmol/l |
| Cholesterol | < 5.2 mmol/l (desirable) |
| | 5.2–6.2 mmol/l (borderline) |
| | > 6.2 mmol/l (high) |
| Serum albumin | 35–55g/l |

NB  'Normal ranges' may vary slightly in different texts.

## Metric measures, units and SI symbols

| Name | SI unit | Symbol |
|---|---|---|
| Mass | gram | g |
| Volume | litre | l |
| Amount of substance | mole | mol |

Standard prefixes are used for decimal submultiples of the units.

| Submultiple | Prefix | Symbol |
|---|---|---|
| $10^{-1}$ | deci- | d |
| $10^{-2}$ | centi- | c |
| $10^{-3}$ | milli- | m |
| $10^{-6}$ | micro- | |
| $10^{-9}$ | nano- | n |
| $10^{-12}$ | pico- | p |

Blood tests may be done before surgery to detect any abnormality that may influence the success of an operation and recovery. For example, if a person is anaemic, their ability to transport oxygen around the body may be lower and they will need to be treated for this condition before surgery. If the surgery is an emergency, a blood transfusion may even be necessary to correct the anaemia.

## Blood glucose estimation

Diseases that involve the breakdown of food and its subsequent use in the body produce energy can be diagnosed by assessing the blood glucose level in the bloo. The level of glucose is maintained by the action of the hormones insulin an glucagon (see Chapter 1). Glucagon enables the body's stores of glucose to b released when needed. Insulin enables the body to store excess glucose as glycogen.

## Changes in blood glucose level

An increase of glucose in the blood may be found in several conditions, the mo important of which is diabetes mellitus. Other conditions include being overweigh inflammation of the pancreas (pancreatitis), tumours of the pancreas and over activ ty of the thyroid gland, thyrotoxicosis.

Similarly, a decreased blood glucose level has many causes. These include exce sive insulin production or administration of insulin, underactivity of the thyroi gland and certain liver diseases.

Some drugs may increase or decrease the blood sugar level. For example, steroi drugs, which may be used to control allergic conditions or inflammation, may cause rise in blood glucose level. Aspirin, used commonly as a pain killer or anticoagulan reduces the blood glucose level.

> **Care point**
>
> A client who has been prescribed steroids for a period of time, for example prednisilone for asthma or chronic bronchitis, will have their urine tested daily for glucose. If there is glucose in their urine, their drug treatment may need to be reviewed.

## Fasting blood glucose estimation

The level of glucose in the blood after a period of approximately eight hours' fastin is a fasting blood glucose level. This investigation is done in the laboratory. Norma fasting blood glucose level is 3.6–5.6 millimoles per litre in adults and 2.2–5.6 mi limoles per litre in children. A result with levels greater than 7.8 millimoles per litr on two or more occasions is sufficient for the diagnosis of diabetes mellitus.

Blood glucose levels may be estimated without the hospital laboratory, using simple finger prick method. This may be used by the diabetic client themselves a home. It is also used by nurses, both in the community and in hospital. A small lanc is used to prick the finger and a large drop of blood allowed to fall onto a speciall impregnated paper. After a set period of time, the paper will have changed colou The change can be compared to a chart which shows blood glucose levels accordin to colour change.

### Cholesterol

**Cholesterol** is often monitored in the blood because raised levels may be associate with the current high incidence of coronary heart disease.

Cholesterol forms the basis of steroid hormones in the body and also the digestiv juice known as bile. Some foods are high in cholesterol (prawns, for example, or egg but the liver also makes cholesterol from animal fat (otherwise known as saturate fat).

The normal cholesterol level in the blood is 3.9–7.2 millimoles per litre. Althoug 'normal', these levels are not ideal and cholesterol levels are, on average, too high in Britain. Levels can rise in conditions that block the flow of bile, or fall in the case of liver diseases, but they are also influenced by the foods we eat. A diet high in animal fats is likely to lead to a high cholesterol level in the blood. In countries where there is a low level of cholesterol in the population, in Japan, for example, the incidence of coronary heart disease is minimal.

**Care point**

> *The Health of the Nation* (see Chapter 6) emphasises the need for a reduction of heart disease in Britain. One of the ways to achieve this is by dietary change and those involved in health education need to be aware of this. A healthy diet is one that is low in animal fat and fast sugars and that contains fibre. The subject of diet was discussed in Chapter 4, *Food, Diet and Nutrition*.

Some clients may develop atherosclerosis, the deposition of fatty plaques that contain cholesterol, in the walls of their arteries. These plaques may narrow the diameter of the blood vessels and may result in reduced blood supply to vital organs. Strokes (a condition resulting from interruption of blood supply to the the brain) and some heart diseases are associated with the diagnosis of atherosclerosis.

**Care point**

> A history of high cholesterol levels in a client is an identified risk factor for the development of coronary heart disease. Review of the diet to reduce the intake of animal fats may play some part in the prevention of heart disease.

## Serum cholesterol measurement

Estimation of the level of cholesterol in the blood, serum cholesterol, may be obtained by a blood sample. This test may be required for clients who develop gall stones or a yellowish staining of the skin (jaundice). The test should also be done as a screening measure for those with raised blood pressure. You may have seen mobile units around shopping centres that will estimate your cholesterol level for a fee.

Any infection of the liver that results in damage to the liver cells will affect their ability to make cholesterol. This will cause a decrease in serum cholesterol level. Cirrhosis of the liver, a chronic disease with widespread destruction of the cells, can cause a low serum cholesterol level. This condition is often a result of alcoholism.

## Blood grouping

There are different systems used to identify the blood type of all humans. The most commonly used systems are the ABO and Rhesus (Rh) systems. Blood type is grouped according to the presence or absence of substances known as antigens (see Chapter 1). Antigens are inherited and are present on most cell membranes, particularly the membrane of the red blood cell. Antigens serve to stimulate the formation of antibodies should they come into contact with unfamiliar potentially harmful substances.

Using the ABO system, the antigens are known as antigen A and antigen B. The absence of antigens is represented by the letter O. Therefore an individual belongs to Group A, Group B, Group AB or Group O. If the blood group is O, there are no antigens on the membrane of the red blood cells. If the blood group is AB, there are bot antigen A and antigen B on the membrane of the red cells.

The plasma does not normally contain antibodies that would react against the ant gens present on its own red cell membrane. This means that Group A would not cor tain antibody a, Group B would not contain antibody b, Group AB would contain n antibodies and Group O would contain both antibody a and antibody b. This i shown in the table below.

## Summary of the ABO system

| Blood group | Red cell antigens | Antibodies in serum | Can donate to groups | Can receive from group |
|---|---|---|---|---|
| AB | A and B | None | AB | All groups |
| A | A | b | A and AB | A and O |
| B | B | a | B and AB | B and O |
| O | None | a and b | All groups | O |

To ascertain an individual's blood group, a sample of his red cells are placed agains a known serum and the reaction is noted. If an antigen causes a reaction to the adde serum, then the term **agglutination**, or clumping, is used to describe the reaction.

## Agglutination when different antibodies are added to blood groups

| Blood group | Serum | | Reaction |
|---|---|---|---|
| | Antibody A | Antibody B | |
| A<br>Antigen A | | | Agglutinates with antibody a |
| B<br>Antigen B | | | Agglutinates with antibody b |
| AB<br>Antigens A and B | | | Agglutinates with both antibody a and antibody b |
| O<br>No antigens | | | No reaction |

- If a person's blood cells agglutinate when mixed with serum that contains antibod a, their blood is Group A.
- If serum containing antibody b agglutinates when in contact with red cells, the antigen B is present and the blood is Group B.
- Group AB shows agglutination when mixed with serum containing antibody a an antibody b.
- Group O shows no evidence of agglutination.

It is necessary to check the blood group before a blood transfusion because if the red cells agglutinate, fragments may travel in the circulation, block small blood vessels in the lungs, heart, brain or kidneys and destroy dependent tissue.

**Care point**

A client who is having a blood transfusion may react adversely to the blood being given. Care must be taken to ensure that the blood groups of the donor and the recipient are compatible In hospitals blood is always checked by two nurses before it is given.

### The Rhesus system

The Rhesus system is indicated by the presence of a D antigen on the red cell membrane. The absence of the D antigen is termed Rhesus negative. The current reference to this system is Rhesus+ve (positive) and Rhesus-ve (negative).

85 per cent of the population in Britain do have the Rhesus antigen and are Rhesus+ve, 15 per cent are Rhesus-ve and do not have the D antigen. Should a Rhesus-ve person be given Rhesus+ve blood, he will make antibodies to the **Rhesus factor**.

In an emergency, the identical blood group may not be available. An individual could receive blood from another group that is least likely to cause an adverse reaction. Group O would be used, as this does not contain either antigen A or antigen B. Group O is known as the 'universal donor'.

Crossmatching samples of blood from donor and recipient helps to reduce incompatibility, the incidence of adverse reactions. In the laboratory the donor red blood cells are exposed to the recipient's plasma to detect other possible cross-reactions.

# The microscopic study of cells

Further direct investigations of body structure and function may be recommended or appropriate in some diseases. Body cells can be examined in more detail than is possible with the naked eye if a section is taken and examined under a microscope. The study under the microscope of the structure, function and disease changes of the body is **histology**.

# Biopsy

The removal of a section of tissue for microscopic investigation is called a biopsy. Biopsy of the liver, kidney or muscle may be carried out to detect changes associated with cancer (cancer cells may also be seen in body secretions, for example in sputum in the case of lung cancer). Other common sites for biopsy include the lung, bone and skin. Biopsies may be obtained through **aspiration** (see page 112) of the cells by a needle or during an operation.

### Liver biopsy

A liver biopsy is performed when liver disease is suspected but is not confirmed by blood tests. It may be to determine the extent of liver damage due to a reaction to drugs, to confirm a suspected tumour or the cause of unexplained jaundice (a yellow coloration of the skin often found in liver disease). As the liver is an organ with a very rich blood supply, certain tests to exclude bleeding tendencies should be carried out prior to the biopsy.

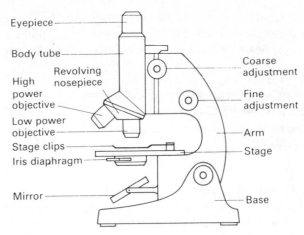

The eyepiece, body tube, revolving nosepiece, high power objective, low power objective, stage clips, iris diaphragm, mirror, coarse adjustment, fine adjustment, arm, stage, base.

*The parts of a microscope*

<table>
</table>

**Care point** — A client with cirrhosis of the liver might require a liver biopsy to determine the cause and extent of the liver damage. It is important that the client lies still during the procedure to prevent the needle slipping and increasing the likelihood of bleeding.

### Kidney biopsy

A kidney biopsy may be used to reveal the pattern of disease changes in the kidneys which may have no known cause and may be due to tumours or progressive kidney failure. A sample of kidney tissue is obtained using a similar method to that for liver biopsy. This test is performed only to obtain information not available from other tests. The location of the kidneys is established before the test by means of an X-ray so that the biopsy needle can be introduced at the correct angle.

**Care point** — After-care advice following a kidney biopsy should include avoiding activities that may cause the kidney to bleed, for example sports or lifting heavy objects.

### Muscle biopsy

A muscle biopsy involves obtaining a sample of tissue usually from the arm or lower leg. This test is used to diagnose conditions or diseases that affect the strength of the muscles and cause them to become smaller (atrophy), for example muscular dystrophy. (Muscular dystrophy is a condition that runs in families and normally affects certain muscle groups. The muscles become atrophied, wasted and weak. There may be deformities of the skeletal framework as a result of the muscles contracting and pulling on the bones to which they are attached. These conditions can affect any age group; children of about five are the largest group, but they may be in adolescence or young adulthood when the condition is suspected.In some cases muscular dystrophy progresses slowly and the individual can still live an active and independent life with few restrictions.)

## Identification of bacteria and viruses

As we have already seen in Chapter 3, some bacteria live inside the body and cause no harm if they remain within their normal habitat. However, some bacteria may attack the tissues and cause disease. The body reacts to the presence of bacteria and viruses by its production of antibodies to protect itself.

The level of antibodies is measured by its strength. This measurement is referred to as the titre. Current infections show a rise in the titre level, while a past incidence shows no change in this level.

The most common bacterial infections are caused by two groups of bacteria, streptococci and staphylococci.

## Streptococci

Streptococci can be found in the throat and other parts of the respiratory system. They can cause diseases such as tonsillitis, meningitis, pneumonia, acute nephritis, wound infections and bacterial endocarditis.

To identify the specific streptococci causing the infection, a swab is taken from the local site, if it is accessible. The laboratory carries out a culture and sensitivity test (see page 110). The end result should identify the streptococci present and the antibiotic treatment that would be effective in the treatment of the infection.

The specimen collected for culture and sensitivity tests may undergo a **Gram stain** in the laboratory. This procedure helps to classify the bacteria by the colour of the dye it retains; it will be known as Gram-positive or Gram-negative. The result narrows down the possible invading bacteria to one of the groups to which they belong and enables antibiotic treatment to start before the final results of the culture are obtained and the exact type of bacteria is known.

Another test that may be used to identify bacteria is an anti-streptococcal antibody test. This test may be used as an alternative when swabs are not possible. The result of the test confirms the presence of streptococci through a blood sample. The response to treatment can also be monitored by the titre level.

**Care point** ▶ When a client requires the collection of a specimen for laboratory examination it is important that the specimen is not contaminated and that it is correctly labelled. The specimen should be placed directly into a sterile container from the laboratory and labelled with the client's full name, age and reference number, if there is one.

## Staphylococci

Staphylococci can also be the cause of many diseases, such as boils, carbuncles, abscesses, wound infections, cystitis, pneumonia and food poisoning. In these cases a culture and sensitivity test is also used to confirm the presence of staphylococci and establish the most appropriate antibiotic treatment. Specimens may be obtained from blood, urine, faeces, sputum and other body fluids.

# Viruses

Some viruses infect a particular cell because of the presence of specific receptors on the cell membrane. Other viruses remain in the host for a time after the original infection. Some diseases caused by viruses are influenza, measles, mumps, rubella, chicken pox, poliomyelitis and meningitis. Adenoviruses found in the adenoids of children can cause many respiratory infections.

A serology test will detect special viral antibodies. This involves the collection of a blood sample. Viral antibody tests confirm exposure to a virus, identify carriers of the virus who may not show symptoms of the infection and ascertain the level of immunity.

### Blood culture

A client with a history of sudden rise in temperature and feeling generally unwell may be recommended for a test to confirm septicaemia. This test to identify the bacteria or viruses causing septicaemia is a blood culture. The test involves the collection of three blood samples in special mediums within a 24-hour period. The samples are generally taken at thirty minute intervals.

**Care point** ▶ A specimen should be obtained from the client and then antibiotic treatment may start before the detailed result is known. It is important that treatment should not begin before the first specimen for culture is obtained; if it does, the bacteria may already be killed and a diagnosis will not be possible. If antibiotic treatment does begin before diagnosis, this should be identified on the laboratory form that accompanies the specimen.

**Activity 7.1**

Visit your doctor's surgery and see the practice nurse there. Ask if you may carry out a survey of the common types and uses of blood tests and other investigations used in the practice. Find out the reasons for doing them and what the normal levels are.

## Screening services

Screening tests are simple tests carried out on a large number of apparently healthy people in order to identify those who may have a specified disease. One example of a screening test is cervical cytology: women may attend their GP or clinic for a smear test; a sample of cells is removed from the cervix and sent to a laboratory to be stained and examined (see also page 127). Cells that are cancerous or overactive and perhaps likely to become cancerous can be detected. Women at risk can be treated before the disease becomes locally invasive or begins to spread around the body.

To be suitable for screening tests a disease should:
- have a high rate of occurrence in the population
- be treatable if detected
- be dangerous if undetected
- be reasonably easy and inexpensive to diagnose at an early stage.

### Disease prevention

The emphasis in health care is increasingly on disease prevention. *Primary Health Care: An Agenda for Discussion* was launched by the Government in April 1986. This comprehensive review of primary health care acknowledged the service of general practitioners in the prevention of ill-health and the promotion of good health. The emphasis was placed on the increasing scope for doing more in early detection of disease. There was a shift in emphasis from an illness service to a health service with the aim of helping to prevent disease and disability. Here are some figures for diseases that could be prevented with more health education and a change in lifestyle:

- 180 000 deaths occur each year from coronary heart disease and 38 million working days are lost
- most women who die from cervical cancer have never had a cervical smear test
- 100 000 deaths are caused by smoking
- 500 million working days are lost and the cost to the NHS for treatment for smoking-related diseases is estimated in the region of £400 million.

Some general practitioners have set up health promotion clinics, manned by practice nurses, in an attempt to decrease incidence of preventable illness. Some screening services are supplied to detect early disease and a change in lifestyle such as stopping smoking or altering the diet may be advised.

In response to *The Health of the Nation*, the government has set targets for health professionals and the public. The aim for the years 1988–2000 is a 30 per cent reduction in deaths of people under 65 from coronary heart disease.

## Activity 7.2

Use your existing knowledge and library resources to investigate changes in lifestyle that you could recommend to a client to reduce their risk of coronary heart disease. Is there any research to support the belief that these changes will influence the rate of occurrence of this disease in the UK?

Another disorder that meets all the requirements for a screening programme is hypertension (high blood pressure).

## Blood pressure measurement

Blood pressure is the amount of pressure that the blood exerts on the walls of the blood vessels as it flows through them. It is an important measurement as it can give important clues as to the state of a person's arteries and is often the first sign of cardiovascular disease. The pressure is measured in millimetres of mercury (mm Hg) using a sphygmomanometer (see overleaf).

Blood pressure varies with age, sex, weight, race, socio-economic status, mood changes, posture, physical activity and general health status. It is lowest in neonates and increases with age, weight gain, stress and anxiety. Shock, myocardial infarction (heart attack), and haemorrhage (blood loss), cause blood pressure to drop below the normal level.

Blood pressure is recorded as two figures. The upper figure, the systolic, is the pressure in the blood vessels as the heart contracts. The lower figure, the diastolic, is the pressure in the vessels when the heart is relaxing between beats. In healthy adults at rest, systolic blood pressure varies between 110 and 140 mm Hg, and diastolic pressure between 75 and 80 mm Hg.

High blood pressure, hypertension, is a risk factor for cardiovascular disease, including coronary heart disease and stroke. Blood pressure is measured during routine health check ups. Life insurance statistics and other research have shown that mortality increases steadily with an increase in blood pressure. About one third of the British population over fifty have raised blood pressure; it is believed that if these people were detected and their blood pressure returned to normal limits the incidence of stroke would be reduced by about 30 per cent.

## Activity 7.3

If blood pressure is only slightly raised, the doctor will not want to prescribe drugs. Rather the client will be persuaded to change their lifestyle. What advice would you give to such a client? Consider, among other influences, which factors in the diet would be important.

### Recording blood pressure

The two pieces of equipment used to record blood pressure are:
- a sphygmomanometer (a cuff which encloses an inflatable rubber bladder)
- a stethoscope.

The most common way to record blood pressure is as follows.

The bell of the stethoscope is placed over the brachial artery. The sphygmomanometer is applied to the arm above the antecubital fossa (elbow). The cuff is inflated and mercury rises up the manometer, from which the pressure is read. The cuff is inflated to approximately 20–30 mm Hg above the last recorded reading, or until the pulse can no longer be heard or palpated. There is a control valve to deflate the system. The pressure valve on the cuff should be released slowly.

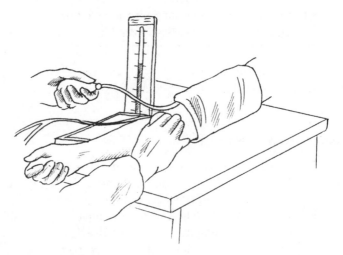

*Measuring blood pressure*

Another method of recording blood pressure is the direct method. A cannula is inserted (by a doctor) into an artery and attached to a pressure-sensitive device. The transmission of a wave form is displayed digitally on a monitor.

**Care point**

It is important to use the correct size of cuff to check blood pressure. There are smaller cuffs available for children. If the wrong size is used, the recording will be inaccurate .

## Respiratory function tests

Ventilation, the process of moving air into and out of the lungs, varies widely with body size, age, and sex. (The effects of exercise on respiration were discussed in Chapter 5.) The vital capacity (VC) is the volume of air expelled by fully breathing out after fully breathing in. It can be measured by a spirometer.

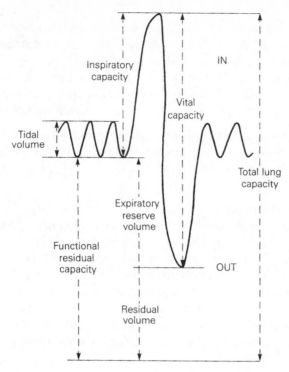

*A spirometer recording*

## Cervical screening

Although the precise cause of cancer is still not known, the risk of cervical cancer is closely related to sexual habits. First intercourse at an early age and multiple partners are considered high risk factors, as is having a large number of sexual contacts.

Cervical cancer screening can prevent development of an invasive cancer. Early detec-tion and prompt treatment mean that there is a good chance of complete recovery. In 1988 the United Kingdom introduced a systematic call-and-recall system, whereby the GP notifies clients by post when a smear is due and when they are due for another one.

The NHS Cervical Screening Programme National Co-ordinating Network, run by district and regional health authorities, have made smear tests available at family planning clinics, general practices and through private consultations with specialists. All women aged between 20 and 64 who are or ever have been sexually active should have a smear test at least every five years. Women who have had an abnormal smear or have been treated for cervical lesions require more frequent smears. The test is taken by scraping cells from the cervix, where any changes begin. An Aylesbury spat-ula is used to obtain the sample.

Results, whether normal or abnormal, are usually conveyed to the woman con-cerned in writing. Women who need referral for treatment should be given an early appointment with their family doctor, to discuss the implications and results.

## Breast screening

Every year there are 26 000 new cases of breast cancer in the UK, of which nearly 16 000 are fatal. The Forest Report (1986) made recommendations which provide a challenge to the primary health care team.

- All women aged between 50 and 64 should be invited for mammography.
- Women aged 65 and over will have mammography on request.
- Women under 50, however, will not be offered routine mammography.

Breast cancer screening is designed to detect invasive cancer at an early stage. The success of such programmes depends on high participation of the target population and an efficient service.

### Testicular cancer

Testicular cancer is the commonest cause of cancer among young men in the UK, accounting for 16 per cent of all cancers in men between the ages of 20 and 44. The majority of cases occur in men between 30 and 34. Although the incidence has increased over the past 15 years, mortality rates have fallen, which is thought to be due to improvements in treatments available.

Early diagnosis is essential. 90 per cent of clients first go to the doctor with a swelling of the testes. Delay in diagnosis is usually caused by embarrassment, fear or lack of awareness that the symptoms can develop into a potentially serious disease.

### Is screening universally beneficial?

Screening for cancer means subjecting large numbers of healthy people to medical procedures for which the vast majority will receive no benefit. Some screening procedures may actually cause harm. The growth rate in most cancers is variable. It is unlikely that screening may benefit all cases. For example, screening the whole adult population for lung cancer by chest X-ray increased the diagnosis levels of the disease but failed to increase the life span of those diagnosed. This screening procedure has therefore been abandoned. In this case, education is likely to be more effective than screening: smoking is strongly correlated to the incidence of lung cancer, so the best advice to the public is to stop smoking. Indeed, health education should aim to stop people from ever starting to smoke.

**Care point**

Carers involved with the screening process should:
- provide clear written information at all stages of the screening process
- have some phone numbers to give to the client, so they can discuss any problems. A client may need some sympathetic support.

Mass screening of the healthy population is becoming an increasingly important part of preventive medicine, although it should not be undertaken unless it is reasonably certain to be effective in reducing the burden of disease. The most important human cost is to the patient. False reassurance causes unnecessary anxiety for the person, their family and friends. Before screening programmes are implemented, resources must be available for treatment and follow-up. The quality of the screening programmes must be sustainable. There is very good evidence that screening for cervical cancer and breast cancer is effective in reducing the long-term mortality. Efficient screening of the population could save many lives.

**Activity 7.2**

For early and accurate diagnosis of disease it is essential that all the services described above are available in the local community and that a good working relationship exists between the various departments involved.

Carry out a survey in your local community of the diagnostic and screening services available. A good place to start may be at your general practitioner's surgery; the practice nurse may tell you which screening services they offer and provide literature to help in your study.

Look at the services offered to, for example, the young, the elderly and expectant mothers. Summarise the role of the component services. Is there good communication between the various departments involved? What do you recommend as improvement to the system?

This work could take the form of a project to be continued throughout your course.

## Twenty questions

1 Give four reasons why it may be necessary to perform blood tests on a client.

2 What is pathology?

3 How would you ensure that a urine specimen to go to the laboratory is as clean as possible?

4 What does the term acid-fast bacillus mean?

5 What is cerebrospinal fluid and where is it found?

6 What is a spirometer used for?

7 What is vital capacity and how may it be measured?

8 Ultrasound is considered to be safer than ordinary X-rays. Why is this?

9 What does an electrocardiogram measure?

10 In what common condition is the blood glucose level raised?

11 For what disease process is raised cholesterol level in the blood considered to be a risk factor?

12 What foods would need to be reduced in an attempt to lower the cholesterol level?

13 What is atherosclerosis?

14 Name the four main blood groups.

15 Which antibodies are attached to the red cell in a person who is blood group O?

16 Name the blood group that is sometimes called 'the universal donor'.

17 Why do we crossmatch blood?

18 Define the term *blood pressure*.

**19** Why do we use screening?

**20** Name two common disease processes that screening may help to eliminate at an early stage.

## Quick concepts

| | |
|---|---|
| **Acid-fast bacillus** | Bacteria that hold their stain after treatment with acid, for example the tubercle bacillus that causes tuberculosis |
| **Angiogram** | An X-ray examination of blood vessels using a dye that is opaque to X-rays |
| **Agglutination** | Sticking together of antigen antibodies to form visible clumps |
| **Aspiration** | Withdrawal by suction of fluid from the body |
| **Audiogram** | Graphic record of a hearing test |
| **Biochemistry** | The study of the chemical processes occurring in living things |
| **Cholesterol** | A steroid lipid implicated in coronary heart disease |
| **Computerised tomography** | Recording 'slices' of an organ by X-ray to see it in more detail |
| **Electrocardiograph** | Tracing of the electrical activity of the heart as measured from the surface of the body |
| **Gram stain** | Method of staining bacterial stains used for identifying different types of bacteria |
| **Haematology** | The study of blood and associated diseases |
| **Histology** | Study of tissues using staining techniques and a microscope |
| **Immunological status** | The presence or absence of antibodies against a specific disease |
| **Mammography** | X-ray photographs of the breast, taken to detect early cancer |
| **Microbiology** | Study of micro-organisms such as bacteria and viruses |
| **Pathology** | Study of disease processes to understand their causes |
| **Phlebotomy** | Puncturing a vein to remove blood |
| **Rhesus factor** | An antigen present on the red cells of 85% of the population |
| **Serology** | Study of the fluid component of the blood |
| **Spirometry** | Tests of ventilation, i.e. breathing |

# Index